HORMONES

Imbalance Is A Symptom, Not A Cause

The R.E.S.T.O.R.E. MILA Series Volume 5

Christopher F. Thoma, DC

307 Longevity

Cody, Wyoming

ISBN:978-1-971449-06-7

Published by 307 Longevity

1120 Beck Ave.

Cody, WY 82414

Second Edition: 2026

Medical Disclaimer

The information presented in this book is for educational purposes only and is not intended as medical advice, diagnosis, or treatment. The content should not be used as a substitute for consultation with a qualified healthcare provider.

The patient stories shared throughout this book are composite narratives created from the author's clinical experiences. Names, identifying details, and circumstances have been changed or combined to protect patient privacy. Any resemblance to specific individuals is coincidental. These narratives are presented to illustrate common patterns observed in clinical practice, not to represent actual patients.

Always consult with your physician or other qualified healthcare provider before making changes to your diet, exercise, supplements, or medications. Individual results may vary, and what works for one person may not be appropriate for another.

Dedication

To my patients, who have taught me more than any textbook ever could. Your courage in the face of chronic illness, your persistence when conventional answers failed, and your willingness to partner with me in exploring a different path - this book exists because of you.

To the mentors and colleagues who shaped my understanding of functional medicine and the body's remarkable capacity to heal. Your wisdom lives in these pages.

To Ashley and Autymn, whose dedication to our patients makes everything we do possible. Your care and commitment are woven into every success story in this practice.

And to my family - Jennifer, Casper, and Sadie - who give meaning to all of it. Your patience during late nights of writing, your support through the challenges of building a practice, and your love that sustains me daily. This work is for you, and because of you.

Contents

Preface

Few words in medicine create as much confusion - and as much profit - as "hormones."

Walk into any anti-aging clinic, functional medicine practice, or even conventional doctor's office with complaints of fatigue, weight gain, brain fog, or low libido, and you'll likely hear the same diagnosis: hormone imbalance. The solution follows predictably - testosterone for men, thyroid medication for everyone whose TSH drifts above a certain number. Bioidentical hormones, pellets, creams, injections, patches. The hormone replacement industry has exploded into a multi-billion-dollar enterprise built on a seductively simple promise: your hormones are low, we'll fill the gap with replacements, and you'll feel better.

The latest trend may be the most troubling of all: testosterone therapy for women. Practitioners are now routinely prescribing testosterone to women complaining of fatigue and low libido - symptoms that have dozens of potential causes rooted in terrain dysfunction. I've seen women in my practice with testosterone levels above 400 ng/dL, when normal female testosterone ranges from roughly 15 to 70 ng/dL. These women are walking around with male-level testosterone coursing through their bodies, experiencing side effects from acne to hair loss to voice changes, while the actual cause of their fatigue remains completely unaddressed.

And now there's another player in this game: peptide therapies. Medications like Ozempic, Wegovy, and Mounjaro have exploded onto the scene, promising effortless weight loss and blood sugar control. What most patients don't realize is that these drugs work by flooding the body with synthetic versions of hormones - GLP-1 and GIP - that your gut naturally produces. They're hormone therapy by another name, manipulating your body's signaling systems at supra-physiological levels while doing nothing to address why your natural hormone production and response became dysfunctional in the first place. The pattern is identical: initial dramatic results, followed by dependency, followed by the realization that stopping the medication brings everything crashing back - often worse than before.

And for a while, these approaches often do make you feel better. That's what makes hormone replacement and peptide therapy so compelling - and so dangerous. The initial improvements are real. Energy returns. Mood lifts. Weight drops. Mental clarity sharpens. Patients become evangelists for their protocols, convinced they've found the answer to their chronic health struggles.

Then, slowly, the benefits fade. Doses need adjustments, additional medications are added and side effects emerge. The body that initially responded so well becomes dependent, requiring external hormones because it has further reduced its own production. What started as a solution has become a trap.

I've watched this pattern unfold hundreds of times in my clinical practice. Patients arrive having tried hormone replacement or peptide therapies - sometimes for years - and they're no better off than when they started. Often they're worse. Their bodies have forgotten how to produce and respond to hormones naturally. Their underlying dysfunction has progressed unchecked. They've treated a symptom while the cause continued its destruction.

This book exists because I'm tired of watching the same patterns repeat.

The Question No One Asks

When a patient presents with low testosterone, low thyroid function, disrupted estrogen and progesterone, or metabolic dysfunction driving weight gain, conventional medicine asks a simple question: What's wrong with the numbers? The answer determines the prescription. Low testosterone? Here's a cream or injection - and now that applies to women too. Low thyroid? Here's Levothyroxine. Can't lose weight? Here's Ozempic. Tired and no libido? Let's check your testosterone and give you a pellet.

Functional medicine often does the same thing, just with "bioidentical" hormones and more sophisticated testing. The philosophy remains identical: find what's abnormal, override it with external intervention.

But there's a far more important question that almost no one asks: Why did hormone production and signaling become impaired in the first place?

Your body didn't randomly decide to stop making adequate hormones or stop responding to them properly. Hormone production requires energy - specifically, ATP produced by mitochondria. It requires raw materials - cholesterol, amino acids, vitamins, and minerals. It requires functional signaling - the hypothalamus talking to the pituitary, talking to the target glands, and the gut talking to the brain about satiety and metabolism. It requires healthy receptor function - cells that are actually able to respond to the hormones circulating in your blood. And it requires a terrain free from the chronic inflammation, toxicity, and immune dysfunction that disrupt every step of this process.

When any of these elements fail, hormone imbalances result. But the imbalance isn't the disease - *it's the symptom.* Treating it with replacement or synthetic peptides is like disconnecting a warning light on your dashboard because you don't like the glow. The light goes off but the problem remains.

The MILA Connection

Throughout my previous books in the R.E.S.T.O.R.E. MILA Series, I've explored how three interconnected systems - Mitochondria, Immune, and Lymphatic - form the axis of human health. When this axis functions properly, the body maintains remarkable resilience. When it becomes dysfunctional, chronic disease emerges.

Hormone dysfunction is no exception. In fact, hormones may be the clearest example of how MILA dysfunction manifests in ways that conventional medicine completely misunderstands.

Consider thyroid dysfunction - the most common hormonal complaint I see in practice. Patients are told their thyroid is "sluggish" or "failing" and given a hormone replacement. But why is the thyroid underperforming? Often, chronic inflammation is directly suppressing thyroid function. This is actually a protective mechanism, because when the body is under stress, a slowing metabolism conserves resources. The immune system may be producing antibodies against thyroid tissue, as in Hashimoto's thyroiditis. Mitochondrial dysfunction in thyroid cells reduces their ability to produce hormones. Nutritional deficiencies - selenium, iodine, zinc - deprive the thyroid of essential building blocks. The Toxic Nine foods and environmental toxins directly damage thyroid tissue and disrupt hormone synthesis.

Replace the hormone, and you've addressed none of these underlying issues. The inflammation continues. The immune attack progresses. The mitochondria remain dysfunctional. The terrain remains broken. You've simply masked the symptom while the underlying disease advances.

The same pattern applies to sex hormones, adrenal function, insulin signaling, and the gut hormones that peptide therapies manipulate. MILA dysfunction creates the conditions for hormone imbalance. Hormone imbalance then worsens

MILA dysfunction. The cycle perpetuates until the actual cause is addressed.

The Exceptions That Prove the Rule

I need to be clear about something important; this book is not an absolute condemnation of all hormone therapy. Two hormones in particular - thyroid hormone and insulin - sometimes require replacement even while terrain restoration proceeds.

Thyroid hormone is essential for virtually every metabolic process. When thyroid function falls below a certain threshold, the body simply cannot heal effectively without support. Trying to restore terrain while severely hypothyroid is like trying to rebuild a house with no electricity - theoretically possible, but practically futile.

Similarly, insulin may be necessary in Type 1 diabetes or advanced Type 2 diabetes where beta cell function has significantly declined. Blood sugar must be controlled to prevent acute harm while working on longer-term restoration.

The difference is intention. These hormones, when necessary, are used as support during healing, not as substitutes for healing. The goal remains terrain restoration. The hormone therapy enables that restoration to proceed. Often, as the terrain heals, hormone requirements decrease or become unnecessary entirely.

This stands in stark contrast to the reflexive hormone replacement and peptide prescribing that dominates current practice - testosterone for tired men and now tired women too, estrogen for every menopausal complaint, Ozempic for everyone who wants to lose weight, bioidenticals for anyone whose labs drift outside arbitrary reference ranges. That approach treats hormones as the destination rather than what they actually are: messengers revealing the state of your terrain.

What You'll Learn

This book will take you on a journey through the complex relationship between hormones and terrain. You'll learn how hormones actually work - not just what they do, but how their production, metabolism, and signaling depend on healthy MILA function. You'll understand why hormone deficiencies often represent protective adaptations rather than random failures. You'll discover how nutritional deficiencies, the Toxic Nine, chronic stress, and environmental toxins create the conditions for hormone dysfunction.

You'll also learn why the current craze of peptide therapies - medications like Ozempic and Mounjaro that promise easy weight loss - represent the same flawed thinking as traditional hormone replacement, just with different molecules and better marketing. These drugs manipulate your body's hormonal signaling without addressing why that signaling became dysfunctional, creating the same patterns of dependency and declining effectiveness.

Most importantly, you'll learn what to do about it. The R.E.S.T.O.R.E. MILA protocol provides a systematic approach to terrain restoration that addresses the root causes of hormone dysfunction. Rather than chasing lab values with prescriptions, you'll understand how to create the terrain conditions where your body can produce, metabolize, and respond to hormones the way it was designed.

The patient stories throughout these chapters are drawn from real clinical experiences - names and details changed to protect privacy, but the patterns and transformations are authentic. These are people who were told their hormone problems were permanent, who were prescribed replacement therapy or peptide medications as a lifelong sentence, and who had given up on their bodies ever functioning normally again. They have now found another way.

You can too.

Hormone imbalance is a symptom, not a cause. It's time we started treating it that way.

With hope for your restoration,

Dr. Christopher Thoma

Introduction

Diana was 47 years old when she walked into my office carrying a shopping bag full of supplements and a folder thick with lab results. She lowered herself into the chair with the careful movements of someone who had learned that her body could betray her at any moment.

"I've tried everything," she said, her voice flat with exhaustion. "And I mean everything."

She was not exaggerating. Diana's journey through the hormone replacement maze had begun five years earlier, when perimenopause hit her hard. The fatigue came first. It was a bone-deep exhaustion that no amount of sleep could touch. Then came the brain fog, so thick some days that she could not remember her own phone number. Her libido vanished. Her joints ached. She gained twenty pounds despite eating less than she had in her thirties. Her hair started thinning. Her skin lost its glow. At night she would lie awake for hours with her mind racing. Then she would drag herself through days that felt like wading through wet concrete.

"My doctor said it was just my hormones," Diana continued. "She ran some labs, told me my estrogen was low, and started me on hormone replacement - estrogen patches. I felt better for about two months. Then everything came back, worse than before."

The dose was increased. Progesterone was added. For another few months, Diana felt almost normal. Then the fatigue returned with a vengeance, joined now by mood swings that frightened her husband and children. She went back to her doctor, who referred her to an endocrinologist.

The endocrinologist ran more labs and found that her thyroid was borderline low. Levothyroxine was prescribed. Another brief improvement, followed by another inevitable decline. Her functional medicine doctor suggested her adrenals were fatigued and added DHEA. A naturopath recommended bioidentical hormones - cleaner than what she had been taking, she was told. An anti-aging clinic measured her testosterone and declared it suboptimal for vitality - testosterone cream was prescribed.

"They kept adding things," Diana said, gesturing at the shopping bag. "Estrogen, progesterone, thyroid, DHEA, testosterone. Plus, supplements for adrenal support, supplements for thyroid conversion, supplements for hormone metabolism. I'm taking twenty-three pills every morning and applying three different creams. My bathroom looks like a pharmacy. And I feel worse than I did five years ago when this all started."

She paused, and I saw tears forming in her eyes.

"Last month, my doctor showed me my latest labs. My testosterone level is 387. She said that's great, that's optimal for energy and libido." Diana's voice cracked. "But I looked it up. Normal testosterone for a woman my age is somewhere between

15 and 70. I have more testosterone than some men. And I still have no energy. I still have no libido. But now I'm growing hair on my chin and losing it on my head. My voice is getting deeper. I have acne like a teenager. What is happening to me?"

The Pattern Behind the Problem

Diana's story is heartbreakingly common. I have heard versions of it hundreds of times. The details differ, but the pattern is always the same.

Someone develops symptoms that disrupt their life. They go to a doctor. Labs are run. A hormone is found to be low. Replacement is prescribed. They feel better for a while. Then the symptoms return. The dose is increased, or another hormone is added. Brief improvement, followed by decline. More hormones, more supplements, more interventions. Each one helps temporarily. None of them lasts. And somewhere along the way, the person becomes dependent on a growing list of prescriptions while feeling progressively worse.

The question nobody seems to ask is: why did the hormones become imbalanced in the first place?

This is not a minor oversight. *It is a fundamental failure in how we think about hormones.* We have been taught to see hormone imbalance as the problem itself - a deficiency to be corrected, a level to be optimized, a number to be normalized. Low estrogen? Add estrogen. Low thyroid? Add thyroid hormone. Low testosterone? Add testosterone. The logic seems straightforward.

But the logic is wrong, and patients like Diana are paying the price.

What This Book Will Teach You

This book rests on a simple but powerful idea: hormone imbalance is almost always a symptom, not a cause. Your hormones did not randomly decide to stop working properly. Something caused them to become imbalanced. And until you address that something, no amount of hormone replacement will create lasting health.

That something is your terrain - the internal environment in which your hormones are produced, transported, received by cells, and cleared from your body. When the terrain is healthy, hormone balance tends to follow naturally. When the terrain is sick, hormones become imbalanced as a downstream consequence. Replacing the hormones without fixing the terrain is like putting fresh oil in an engine that is overheating. You have addressed a symptom while ignoring the actual problem.

The Terrain That Determines Everything

What do I mean by terrain? Think of your body as a garden. The hormones are like the plants you want to grow. But plants do not grow in isolation. They need soil with the right nutrients. They need adequate water and sunlight. They need protection from pests and disease. They need proper drainage, so their roots do not rot. You can plant the most beautiful seeds in the world, but if the soil is toxic, the drainage is blocked, and pests are everywhere, those plants will never thrive.

Your hormones work the same way. They depend on a healthy internal environment to function properly. That environment is shaped by three interconnected systems that I call the MILA axis: your Mitochondria, your Immune system, and your Lymphatic system.[2]

Your mitochondria are the tiny power plants inside your cells. They produce the energy your body needs for everything it does - including making hormones. Hormone production is energy-expensive work.[3] The conversion of cholesterol into pregnenolone, the mother hormone from which all steroid hormones are made, requires substantial energy in the form of ATP. When your mitochondria are struggling, they cannot provide enough energy for optimal hormone production. No amount of hormone replacement can override this fundamental energy deficit.

Your immune system does far more than fight infections. It regulates inflammation throughout your body, and inflammation directly affects hormone function.[4] Chronic low-grade inflammation - the kind caused by poor diet, gut dysfunction, hidden infections, and toxic exposures - suppresses hormone production. It impairs the conversion of inactive hormones to their active forms. It damages the receptors that allow cells to receive hormone signals. An overactive or dysregulated immune system is one of the most common causes of hormone dysfunction.

Your lymphatic system is your body's drainage network. It removes waste products, excess fluid, and used hormones from your tissues.[5] When the lymphatic system becomes congested - from sedentary lifestyle, chronic inflammation, or inadequate hydration - hormone metabolites accumulate in your tissues. This can create imbalances that look like deficiencies but are actually clearance problems. You might not need more hormones. You might just need to clear the ones that have built up.

These three systems - mitochondria, immune, and lymphatic - form an axis. I list them in that order for a reason. Mitochondrial dysfunction is at the root of most chronic diseases in the human body.[6] When your mitochondria fail, everything downstream fails with them. Immune dysfunction comes next - when the immune system becomes dysregulated, it creates inflammation that damages tissues and disrupts signaling throughout the body. Lymphatic stagnation follows - when drainage fails, toxins and waste products accumulate, making everything worse.

But here is something critical to understand: while mitochondrial dysfunction may be the deepest root of the problem, you cannot start treatment there. If you try to supercharge damaged mitochondria while the lymphatic system is clogged and the immune system is in chaos, you will make things worse. You will mobilize toxins that cannot be cleared. You will increase energy production in a system that is already inflamed and overwhelmed.

This is why the R.E.S.T.O.R.E. MILA protocol works in reverse order. We start by opening drainage pathways and supporting lymphatic flow. Then we calm down and regulate the immune system. Only after the terrain can properly clear waste and inflammation has been brought under control do we address mitochondrial function directly. This sequence is not optional. It is essential for safe and successful restoration of health.

When the MILA axis works well together, your terrain is healthy and your hormones tend to balance naturally. When any of these systems become dysfunctional, the whole system suffers. And critically, this axis has a two-way relationship with your hormones. Unhealthy terrain causes hormone dysfunction, but hormone dysfunction also damages the terrain. It becomes a vicious cycle that keeps getting worse until someone addresses the root cause in the right order.

What Damages the Terrain

If the terrain is so important, what damages it in the first place? In my clinical experience, a few factors come up again and again.

The first factor is what I call the Toxic Nine - a group of foods that cause inflammation and gut dysfunction in a large percentage of people. These are sugar, wheat and gluten, corn, soy, dairy, peanuts, seed oils, alcohol, and chemical additives. Not everyone reacts to all of them. But most people with chronic health issues are reacting to at least some of them, often without realizing it. These foods damage the gut lining, trigger immune activation, and create the chronic inflammation that disrupts hormone function.

The second factor is omega fatty acid imbalance. Your cell membranes - the outer walls of every cell in your body, including the cells that produce and respond to hormones - are made largely of fatty acids. The modern diet has dramatically shifted the ratio of omega-6 to omega-3 fats, often reaching 18 to 1 or higher when it should be closer to 2 to 1. This imbalance makes cell membranes rigid and dysfunctional. Hormone receptors embedded in those membranes cannot work properly. Cells cannot receive hormone signals even when the hormones are present in adequate amounts.

The third factor is toxic exposure. We are surrounded by chemicals that directly interfere with hormone function - in our food, our water, our personal care products, our household cleaners, even the receipts we handle at the grocery store.[6] These endocrine disruptors can mimic hormones, block hormone receptors, and interfere with hormone production and metabolism. They accumulate in our tissues over time, creating an increasing burden on the MILA axis.

The fourth factor is chronic stress. When your body perceives threat - whether from a physical danger, financial worry, relationship conflict, or just the relentless pace of modern life - it prioritizes survival over everything else.[8] Resources get shunted toward stress hormones and away from sex hormones and thyroid function. This makes sense as a short-term survival strategy. But when stress never lets up, the system stays stuck in survival mode indefinitely.

Why Replacement Fails

Understanding the terrain helps explain why hormone replacement so often fails - and why it can actually make things worse.

When you add hormones from outside, you do nothing to fix the damaged terrain. The mitochondria are still struggling. The inflammation is still present. The lymphatic congestion remains. The toxic burden has not changed. You have added hormones to a system that cannot use them properly. It is like pouring more water into a clogged drain.

Worse, the external hormones trigger your body's feedback systems. Your brain senses the increased hormone levels and concludes that it can reduce its own internal hormone signals telling your glands to reduce hormone production.[9] Over time, your natural hormone production drops even further. Your glands, no longer being asked to work, can actually shrink. Now you are dependent on external hormones because your body has partially lost the ability to make its own.

This explains the pattern Diana experienced: initial improvement followed by decline, requiring ever-increasing doses or additional hormones. The replacement provided temporary relief while the underlying terrain continued to deteriorate.

Eventually, even high doses could not overcome a body that was too inflamed, too toxic, and too exhausted to respond properly.

And then there is the problem of supra-physiological dosing - providing hormone levels far above what the body would naturally produce. Diana's testosterone at 387 ng/dL was five to twenty times higher than would be expected for a healthy woman her age. While this might temporarily improve energy or libido, it creates a cascade of other problems.[10] The body was never designed to run on those levels. The side effects Diana experienced - facial hair growth, scalp hair loss, deepening voice, acne - were her body's response to hormone levels it was never meant to handle.

A Different Path

When I explained all of this to Diana, I watched something shift in her expression. For the first time in years, what was happening to her made sense.

"So, all these hormones I've been taking," she said slowly, "they've been treating the wrong thing?"

"They've been treating a symptom," I replied, "while the actual cause - your terrain - kept getting worse. Your body was trying to tell you something was wrong. Low hormones were the message. Instead of hearing the message and fixing the underlying problem, you were given hormones to cover it up."

"Can it be fixed?" she asked. "After all this time, after all these hormones - can my body actually recover?"

The answer, I told her, was yes - with patience and the right approach.

Over the following months, we worked through the R.E.S.T.O.R.E. MILA protocol. We did not start by removing her hormones - that would have been too abrupt for a body that had become dependent on them. Instead, we focused first on restoring her terrain.[11]

She eliminated the Toxic Nine foods and watched her chronic bloating disappear within weeks. She corrected her omega fatty acid ratio. She supported her lymphatic drainage. She addressed hidden gut infections that had been driving inflammation for years. She reduced her toxic exposures. Step by step, her terrain began to heal.

As her terrain improved, something remarkable happened. Her body began producing its own hormones again. Under careful medical supervision, she was able to gradually reduce her external hormones. Her energy returned - real, sustained energy, not the jittery false energy she had gotten from supra-physiological testosterone. Her brain fog lifted. Her mood stabilized. Her hair stopped falling out. The chin hairs stopped appearing.

Six months after beginning the protocol, Diana sat in my office again. This time she was not carrying a shopping bag of supplements.

"I'm down to three things," she said, smiling. "And my labs look better than they have in five years. But more importantly, I feel like myself again. I didn't realize how much I had lost until I got it back."

You deserve to understand what is happening in your body. You deserve to know why the solutions you have been offered have not worked. And you deserve a path forward that addresses the real problem, not just the symptoms. That is what this book will give you.

But before we can fix what is broken, we need to understand how the system is supposed to work. In the next chapter, we will explore the hormone hierarchy - how your hormones are made, how they communicate with each other, and why treating one hormone in isolation almost always fails. Let's begin.

Key Takeaways

- Hormone imbalance is a symptom of terrain dysfunction, not a disease requiring lifelong replacement.

- The MILA axis - mitochondria, immune, and lymphatic axis - determines whether hormones can be produced and received properly.

- Hormone replacement creates dependency while leaving damaged terrain unaddressed.
- Treatment must address MILA in reverse order - lymphatics first, then immune, then mitochondria.
- Terrain restoration allows the body to resume natural hormone production without permanent dependence.

Chapter 1

The Hormone Hierarchy

What Hormones Actually Are

Before we can understand why hormones become imbalanced, we need to understand what they actually are and how they work. Think of hormones as your body's text messages. They carry instructions from one part of your body to another, telling cells what to do and when to do it.

Your body makes dozens of different hormones, but they fall into a few main categories. Steroid hormones - including cortisol, testosterone, estrogen, and progesterone - are all made from cholesterol. This is important, and we will come back to it. Peptide hormones - like insulin and growth hormone - are made from amino acids, the building blocks of protein. Thyroid hormones are in their own special category, made from the amino acid tyrosine plus iodine.

Each type of hormone works differently. Steroid hormones are fat-soluble, meaning they can pass right through cell membranes and go directly into the cell to affect gene expression.[7] Peptide hormones are water-soluble, so they have to knock on the door by binding to receptors on the outside of the cell. The receptor then passes the message inside. This difference matters because it affects how quickly hormones work and how long their effects last.

The Master Glands: Your Body's Control Center

At the base of your brain sit two tiny glands that run the whole show: the hypothalamus and the pituitary. The hypothalamus is like a thermostat. It constantly monitors hormone levels in your blood and decides whether you need more or less of each one.[12] When it senses that a hormone is low, it sends a signal to the pituitary gland.

The pituitary is often called the master gland because it controls so many other glands throughout your body. When it gets a signal from the hypothalamus, it releases its own hormones that travel through the bloodstream to your thyroid, adrenal glands, ovaries, or testes. Those glands then produce their specific hormones - thyroid hormone, cortisol, testosterone, estrogen, etc.

Here is where it gets interesting. Once those hormones are released, they travel back to the hypothalamus and pituitary. When levels get high enough, they tell those master glands to stop sending signals.[9] This is called negative feedback, and it is how your body keeps hormone levels in a healthy range. It is also why taking hormones from outside can cause problems - but we will get to that.

Cholesterol: The Building Block You Have Been Taught to Fear

For decades, we have been told that cholesterol is the enemy. Lower it at all costs. Take statins. Avoid eggs. But here is what those messages leave out: cholesterol is the raw material your body uses to make every single steroid hormone.[13] Without enough cholesterol, you literally cannot make cortisol, testosterone, estrogen, progesterone, or vitamin D (which is actually a hormone, not a vitamin).[14]

The hormone-making process starts when cholesterol gets converted into something called pregnenolone. This happens inside your mitochondria - the energy factories in your cells - and it takes a lot of energy to do.[15] Right here, at the very first step, we see why mitochondrial health matters so much for hormone health. If your mitochondria are struggling, they cannot efficiently turn cholesterol into pregnenolone, and everything downstream suffers.

Pregnenolone is called the mother hormone because all other steroid hormones come from it.[16] From pregnenolone, the pathway splits. One branch leads to progesterone, and then to cortisol and aldosterone. Another branch leads to DHEA, and from there to testosterone and estrogen.[13] These pathways share the same starting material and compete for the same resources. When your body needs more of one hormone, it often means making less of another. This is not a flaw. It is intelligent resource management.

The Pregnenolone Steal: When Survival Trumps Everything Else

This brings us to something really important: the pregnenolone steal. When your body is under constant stress, it has to make a choice. It can use its raw materials to make stress hormones, or it can use them to make sex hormones. It cannot do both equally well.[12]

Your body will always choose survival first. If it senses danger - and chronic modern stress feels like danger to your biology - it will pour resources into making cortisol.[9] Testosterone, estrogen, and progesterone production drops as a result. This is not a mistake. This is your body being smart. If you were running from a predator, you would not need to reproduce. You would need to survive.

The problem is that modern life keeps this survival switch turned on. Work stress, financial worry, poor sleep, inflammatory foods, hidden infections - your body reads all of these as threats.[8] So it keeps choosing cortisol over sex hormones, day after day, year after year.

Now here is where hormone replacement becomes a problem.

When a doctor sees your low testosterone or low estrogen, they often reach for a prescription. But think about what is actually happening. Your body made a deliberate choice to lower those hormones. It did this because it sensed danger and needed to redirect resources. The low hormone level is not the problem. It is your body's response to a problem.

When you take external hormones, you override that choice. But you have not removed the danger. You have not fixed the stress. You have not restored the energy systems that would allow your body to make enough hormones for everything. You have just forced one number higher on a lab test while everything underneath stays broken.[17]

It gets worse. When you add hormones from outside, your brain notices. It says, we have plenty of testosterone now, so we can stop asking the body to make more. The signals that tell your glands to produce hormones get weaker.[9] Over time, your own production drops even further. Your hormone-producing glands, no longer being asked to work, can actually shrink.

Meanwhile, the original stress continues. Your body still needs cortisol. It still shunts resources away from sex hormones. Now you are dependent on external hormones, your body makes even less of its own than before, and the underlying problem remains completely unaddressed.

This is why so many people describe the same pattern with hormone replacement. They feel better at first - sometimes dramatically better. Then they plateau. Then they start feeling worse again.[18] The external hormone helped with symptoms for a while, but the terrain kept getting sicker. Eventually, even high doses cannot overcome a body that is too inflamed, too toxic, and too exhausted to respond properly.

The same thing happens with every type of hormone replacement. Give thyroid hormone to someone whose real problem is inflammation, blocking hormone activation, and you have not fixed anything. Give estrogen to a woman whose body is in survival mode, and you have masked the signal without hearing the message. Give cortisol to someone whose stress response is broken, and you make the stress response even weaker.[19]

Here is what we need to understand: your body was trying to tell you something. Low testosterone was a message saying the terrain is under threat. Low thyroid was a message saying the system is conserving energy because something is wrong. These were not simply deficiencies to fill. They were warning lights on the dashboard.

When we give hormones without addressing why they dropped, we are covering up the warning light with tape. The light is no longer visible, but the engine is still failing.

The Thyroid: Your Metabolic Thermostat

Your thyroid gland sits at the front of your neck and controls how fast everything in your body runs. It affects how quickly you burn calories, how efficiently your mitochondria produce energy, how fast your heart beats, how well you think, and how effectively you maintain body temperature.[5] When thyroid function is optimal, everything works better. When it is impaired, everything suffers.

The thyroid mainly produces T4, which is actually a storage form of thyroid hormone. T4 has to be converted into T3 to become active.[3] This conversion happens throughout your body, but especially in the liver and gut. It requires selenium, zinc, and adequate energy. Most importantly, it is extremely sensitive to inflammation.

When inflammation is present, your body converts less T4 to active T3 and more to something called reverse T3, which actually blocks T3 from working.[20] This means you can have normal TSH and T4 on your lab tests while being functionally hypothyroid at the cellular level. The T4 is there, but it is not converting to the active form. Or the T3 is there, but reverse T3 is blocking it from doing its job.

This is why so many patients are told their thyroid is fine when they clearly have every symptom of low thyroid function. The standard tests miss the real problem.

Cortisol: The Hormone That Gets Blamed for Everything

Cortisol has gotten a bad reputation as the stress hormone that makes you fat and sick. But cortisol is essential for life. You would die within days without it.[21] The problem is not cortisol itself. The problem is what happens when cortisol production becomes chronically dysregulated.

In a healthy body, cortisol follows a daily rhythm. It peaks in the morning to help you wake up and gradually declines throughout the day, reaching its lowest point at night so you can sleep.[19] Cortisol also spikes in response to acute stress, then returns to normal when the threat passes.

Chronic stress breaks this rhythm. Initially, you may produce too much cortisol all the time - high in the morning, high at night, high when there is no obvious threat. Over time, your adrenal glands can become exhausted, and cortisol production drops too low.[22] Either extreme causes problems, or the pattern often shifts from one to the other as the dysfunction progresses.

What you need to understand is that abnormal cortisol patterns are almost always a symptom of something else - chronic inflammation, gut dysfunction, blood sugar instability, or the overall burden on your terrain. Trying to treat cortisol directly without addressing these underlying factors rarely works for long.

Insulin: The Hormone That Controls the Others

Insulin might be the most important hormone to understand because it affects virtually every other hormone system in your body. Its main job is to move sugar from your blood into your cells, where it can be used for energy.[23] But insulin does much more than that.

When insulin is chronically elevated - a condition called hyperinsulinemia, that often precedes diabetes by years or decades - it disrupts everything. High insulin increases an enzyme called aromatase, which converts testosterone to estrogen.[24] This is why men with insulin resistance often develop low testosterone and why women with insulin resistance often have estrogen dominance. High insulin also promotes cortisol secretion, impairs growth hormone release, and increases inflammatory signals that disrupt thyroid and sex hormone function.

The bottom line is simple: you cannot have healthy hormone function with dysfunctional insulin signaling. Any attempt to balance hormones without addressing insulin resistance is likely to fail.

This is one area where the R.E.S.T.O.R.E. MILA protocol acknowledges that some people may need insulin support - particularly those with Type 1 diabetes, or advanced Type 2 diabetes, where the pancreas can no longer produce adequate insulin. But even then, terrain restoration can often reduce the amount of support needed and prevent further progression.

You may have heard of the new weight loss drugs like Ozempic and Mounjaro. These medications work by mimicking gut hormones called GLP-1 and GIP that affect insulin release and appetite. While they can produce dramatic weight loss, they also come with significant side effects and create their own form of dependence. When people stop taking them, the weight typically returns because the underlying terrain dysfunction was never addressed. We will explore this in more detail in a later chapter.

Sex Hormones: More Than Reproduction

When people think of sex hormones, they think of reproduction. But testosterone, estrogen, and progesterone do far more than regulate fertility. They affect your brain, your bones, your heart, your mood, your energy, and your ability to build and maintain muscle.[10]

Testosterone is essential for both men and women, though in different amounts. Normal testosterone in men ranges from about 300 to 1000 ng/dL. Normal testosterone in women ranges from about 15 to 70 ng/dL.[10] These are dramatically different ranges, and this matters when we discuss testosterone therapy for women later in this book.

Estrogen is not one hormone, but a family of hormones, with estradiol being the most active form. Estrogen protects brain function, maintains bone density, keeps skin elastic, and supports cardiovascular health.[25] Progesterone balances estrogen, supports sleep, calms the nervous system, and is essential for maintaining pregnancy.

When these hormones decline with age, it is tempting to simply replace them. But the question we should be asking is why they declined. Was it purely aging, or was it terrain dysfunction that accelerated the decline? In most cases, it is both - and addressing the terrain can often restore a significant amount of function without creating dependence on external hormones.

There is another issue worth mentioning here. In recent years, testosterone therapy has become increasingly popular for women - not just menopausal women, but younger women complaining of fatigue and low libido. Remember those normal ranges: women naturally have between 15 and 70 ng/dL of testosterone. Yet some clinics are dosing women to levels of 150,

200, or even higher - two to ten times what a healthy woman would naturally produce. The short-term effects may feel good. The long-term consequences of running these supra-physiological levels are still being discovered, and early signs suggest they are not good.

Why Treating One Hormone Never Works

Every hormone affects every other hormone. This is not an exaggeration. Low thyroid function leads to accumulation of estrogen and cortisol because metabolism is too slow to clear them.[26] Cortisol blocks TSH and impairs T4 to T3 conversion, so chronic stress causes functional hypothyroidism even when the thyroid gland itself is fine. Estrogen increases a protein that binds to thyroid hormone, reducing how much is available for use.[27] Each connection creates the potential for cascading dysfunction - or cascading improvement when the terrain is restored.

This interconnection is why treating one hormone in isolation fails so consistently. Give thyroid hormone without addressing cortisol, and you may accelerate an already overtaxed system. Give testosterone without addressing insulin resistance, and much of it converts to estrogen. Give estrogen without progesterone, and you create imbalance. Replace cortisol without fixing the stress response, and you suppress what remains of natural production.[28]

The terrain-based approach recognizes that hormone imbalances do not occur in isolation because hormones do not function in isolation. Restoring the mitochondrial energy production, immune regulation, and lymphatic flow that all hormone systems depend upon creates the conditions for the entire hierarchy to rebalance naturally.

Understanding this hierarchy is the foundation for everything that follows. In the next chapter, we will explore what happens when the terrain breaks down - how mitochondrial dysfunction, immune dysregulation, and lymphatic congestion create the conditions for hormone imbalance, and why the body's intelligent adaptations to this dysfunction are often mistaken for diseases requiring treatment.

Key Takeaways

- Hormones exist in a hierarchy where each one influences and depends upon the others.

- Cholesterol is the essential building block for all steroid hormones, which is why aggressively lowering it can cause hormone problems.

- The pregnenolone steal shunts resources toward cortisol during chronic stress, causing sex hormones to drop as an intelligent survival adaptation.

- Hormone replacement often makes things worse by overriding intelligent adaptations, suppressing natural production, and masking the signals that something deeper is wrong.

- Treating one hormone in isolation fails because hormones never function in isolation - restoring the terrain allows the entire system to rebalance.

Chapter 2

The Terrain That Breaks Down

When the Terrain Breaks

Robert was 52 years old when his doctor told him his testosterone was low. The number on the lab report was 289 ng/dL - just under the 300 that most labs consider the bottom of normal. His doctor pulled out a prescription pad.

"This is why you're tired all the time," his doctor said. "This is why your workouts aren't producing results anymore. This is probably affecting your mood, your focus, maybe even your marriage. Testosterone replacement will change your life."

Robert had heard the ads. Low T. It explained everything. Men his age were supposed to feel this way, and the solution was simple - just add testosterone. His doctor made it sound so straightforward.

But something made Robert pause. His father had started testosterone therapy at about the same age. Initially, it seemed like a miracle. His energy returned and his mood improved. But within two years, his father was on a higher dose, and then later a higher one still. He eventually developed sleep apnea. His prostate enlarged. His body stopped producing its own testosterone entirely, and when he tried to stop the therapy, he crashed hard. At 74, Robert's father was still dependent on testosterone injections, managing side effects with additional medications, and no healthier than when he started.

"Before I start this," Robert said, "I want to understand why my testosterone dropped in the first place. I was fine ten years ago. What changed?"

His doctor looked surprised. Most patients just wanted the prescription. "It's probably just age," he said. "Testosterone naturally declines as men get older."

"But my father's testosterone was fine into his sixties," Robert pressed. "And I know men in their seventies who still have normal levels. There has to be something else going on."

That question - what else is going on - led Robert to my office. And it led to a vastly different outcome than the one his doctor had predicted.

The Question That Changes Everything

Robert asked the question that almost nobody asks: why did my hormones become imbalanced? It seems obvious, but in conventional medicine, this question is almost never explored. The lab value is low, so they replace it. A number is abnormal, so they normalize it. The underlying cause remains a mystery - and more importantly, it remains unaddressed.

When I examined Robert's full history, the picture became clear. Over the past decade, his life had changed dramatically. He had taken a high-stress position at work, regularly sleeping five to six hours instead of eight. He had gained forty pounds, most of it around his midsection. He ate lunch at his desk - usually fast food or something from a vending machine. He had stopped exercising regularly. He drank more than he used to, just to unwind at night. He had developed acid reflux and was taking a proton pump inhibitor daily. He had been on two courses of antibiotics in the past year for sinus infections.

His testosterone had not randomly dropped. His terrain had deteriorated, and his hormones had responded accordingly. His body was doing exactly what it was designed to do when facing chronic stress, inflammation, and metabolic dysfunction - it was conserving resources and prioritizing survival over vitality.

What We Mean by Terrain

The concept of terrain comes from an old debate in medicine. In the late 1800s, two scientists - Louis Pasteur and Antoine Bechamp - argued about what caused disease. Pasteur believed germs were everything. Kill the germ, cure the disease. Bechamp believed the terrain was everything. A healthy internal environment would resist disease; a sick terrain would succumb to it.

History sided with Pasteur, and we got antibiotics and the germ theory of disease. But Bechamp was not entirely wrong. We now know that the same bacteria can live harmlessly in one person and cause severe illness in another. The difference is the terrain - the internal environment that either supports health or creates vulnerability to disease.

When it comes to hormones, terrain is everything. Your hormones do not exist in a vacuum. They are produced by cells that need energy and raw materials. They travel through blood and lymph that must be flowing properly. They deliver their messages to receptors that must be functioning correctly. They are cleared by detoxification pathways that must be working efficiently. When any of these systems breaks down, hormone problems follow.

The Three Pillars of Terrain: The MILA Axis

In my clinical experience, three systems form the foundation of terrain health. I call them the MILA axis: Mitochondria, Immune, and Lymphatic. Understanding how each of these affects' hormone function - and how they interact with each other - is essential for understanding why hormone imbalances develop and how to actually fix them.

Mitochondria: The Energy Crisis at the Root of Everything

Your mitochondria are tiny structures inside almost every cell in your body. Their primary job is to produce energy in the form of ATP - the fuel that powers everything your cells do.[6] You have trillions of mitochondria, and they produce roughly your body weight in ATP every single day. When they are working well, you have abundant energy. When they are struggling, everything suffers.

Hormone production is one of the most energy-demanding processes in your body. The conversion of cholesterol to pregnenolone - the first step in making all steroid hormones - happens inside the mitochondria and requires substantial ATP.[13] If your mitochondria cannot produce enough energy, this conversion slows down. Less pregnenolone means less raw material for testosterone, estrogen, progesterone, cortisol, and all the other steroid hormones.

But mitochondrial dysfunction does not just reduce hormone production. It also triggers something called the Cell Danger Response.[29] When mitochondria sense threat - from toxins, infections, or metabolic stress - they shift from energy production mode to defense mode. They start producing signals that tell the rest of the cell, and indeed the whole body, that danger is present. These signals trigger inflammation, alter metabolism, and fundamentally change how the body allocates resources.

In defense mode, the body prioritizes immediate survival over long-term functions like reproduction and optimal metabolism. Hormone production drops not because something is broken, but because the body is intelligently conserving resources for what it perceives as a crisis. This is why mitochondrial dysfunction is at the root of so many chronic diseases - and why I list it first in the MILA axis.[30]

Immune Dysfunction: When Protection Becomes the Problem

Your immune system is designed to protect you from threats - bacteria, viruses, parasites, and abnormal cells. When it is working properly, it mounts an appropriate response to genuine threats and then calms down when the threat is gone. But in many people with chronic health issues, the immune system has become dysregulated. It is not necessarily weak. Often, it is overactive, stuck in a state of chronic low-grade inflammation.[6]

This chronic inflammation directly interferes with hormone function at multiple levels. Inflammatory cytokines - the chemical messengers of the immune system - suppress the hypothalamus and pituitary, reducing the signals that tell your glands to produce hormones.[31] They impair the enzymes that convert inactive hormones to active forms. They damage hormone receptors, making cells less responsive to the hormones that are present. They even alter how hormones are metabolized and cleared from the body.

Perhaps most importantly, chronic inflammation tells your mitochondria to stay in defense mode. This creates a vicious cycle: inflammation impairs mitochondrial function, and impaired mitochondria produce more inflammatory signals. The terrain becomes progressively more dysfunctional, and hormone imbalances become progressively worse.

What causes chronic immune activation in the first place? The list includes gut dysfunction and intestinal permeability, chronic infections (viral, bacterial, or fungal), food sensitivities (especially to the Toxic Nine), environmental toxin exposure, chronic stress, and blood sugar dysregulation.[32] In Robert's case, his poor diet, disrupted gut function from antibiotics, chronic stress, and excess body fat were all contributing to immune dysregulation.

Lymphatic Stagnation: When the Drainage System Fails

Your lymphatic system is the forgotten component of circulation. While everyone knows about blood flowing through arteries and veins, few people think about lymph - the clear fluid that bathes your tissues, collects waste products, and carries immune cells throughout your body.[33]

Unlike blood, which is pumped by the heart, lymph has no central pump. It relies on muscle movement, breathing, and the gentle pulsing of the lymph vessels themselves to keep flowing. When you are sedentary, dehydrated, or chronically inflamed, lymphatic flow slows dramatically. Waste products accumulate. Immune function becomes impaired. And importantly for our purposes, hormone metabolites - the breakdown products of used hormones - build up in your tissues.

This can create hormone imbalances that look like deficiencies but are actually clearance problems. You might not need more estrogen - you might just need to clear the estrogen metabolites that have accumulated. You might not have a progesterone deficiency - you might have a progesterone that cannot get to its receptors because the interstitial fluid is congested.[34]

Lymphatic stagnation also impairs the immune system, since lymph nodes are where immune cells congregate and coordinate their responses. Poor lymphatic flow means poor immune surveillance, which can allow chronic low-grade infections to persist - infections that further drive inflammation and mitochondrial dysfunction.

Why the Order Matters: You Cannot Start at the Root

I list the MILA axis as Mitochondria, Immune, Lymphatic because that is the order of how deep the dysfunction goes. Mitochondrial problems are at the root - they affect everything else. Immune dysfunction comes next; both causing and being caused by mitochondrial problems. Lymphatic stagnation follows, making both mitochondrial and immune problems worse.

But here is what many practitioners get wrong: *you cannot start treatment at the root.* If you try to directly boost mitochondrial function while the lymphatic system is clogged and the immune system is in overdrive, you will make things worse. You will be adding energy to a system that cannot clear waste properly. You will be revving an engine that is overheating.

This is why the R.E.S.T.O.R.E. MILA protocol works in reverse order. We start by opening drainage pathways and supporting lymphatic flow - making sure waste products can get out. Then we calm and regulate the immune system - reducing the inflammation that is driving so much of the dysfunction. Only after the terrain can properly drain and inflammation is under control do we address mitochondrial function directly.

This sequence is not optional. It is essential for safe and effective restoration. Patients who try to skip steps - or practitioners who go straight to mitochondrial support - often experience what is called a healing crisis: a temporary but sometimes severe worsening of symptoms as toxins are mobilized faster than they can be cleared. The proper sequence avoids this.

What Robert's Terrain Revealed

When we assessed Robert's terrain through the MILA lens, the picture was clear. His mitochondria were struggling - years of poor sleep, high stress, and a heavy diet in the Toxic Nine had taken their toll. His fasting insulin was elevated, a sign that his cells were becoming resistant and his mitochondria were not efficiently burning fuel.[35]

His immune system was dysregulated. His C-reactive protein, a marker of inflammation, was elevated. His gut had been disrupted by antibiotics, and stool testing revealed an overgrowth of opportunistic bacteria along with reduced diversity of beneficial species.[36] His diet was full of inflammatory foods - gluten, dairy, sugar, and seed oils at nearly every meal.

His lymphatic system had become sluggish. He sat at a desk for ten hours a day, rarely exercised, and drank coffee instead of water. He had chronic sinus congestion - a sign of lymphatic stagnation in the head and neck. His legs would swell by the end of the day.

We also found that his omega fatty acid ratio was severely imbalanced. Testing showed a ratio of 22 to 1 omega-6 to omega-3 - far from the ideal of 2 to 1. This meant his cell membranes, including the membranes of the cells that produce and respond to testosterone, were rigid and dysfunctional. His vitamin D level was also low at 24 ng/mL, when optimal is between 50 and 80. Since vitamin D functions as a hormone and is essential for testosterone production, this deficiency was directly contributing to his problem.

In this context, his low testosterone made perfect sense. His body was not making a mistake. It was doing exactly what a body should do when the terrain is this compromised: conserving resources, prioritizing survival, and waiting for conditions to improve before investing in functions like optimal hormone production.

A Different Path

Robert never started testosterone therapy. Instead, he committed to restoring his terrain.

The first step was eliminating the Toxic Nine - sugar, wheat and gluten, corn, soy, dairy, peanuts, seed oils, alcohol, and chemical additives. This alone reduced his inflammatory burden significantly. Within three weeks, his acid reflux had resolved and he was able to stop his proton pump inhibitor. Within six weeks, his energy had noticeably improved and he had lost twelve pounds without trying.

We supported his lymphatic system with simple interventions - daily movement, proper hydration, dry brushing, and specific breathing exercises. We addressed his gut dysfunction with targeted probiotics and gut-healing nutrients. We supported his sleep, gradually extending his nights from five hours to seven.

We corrected his omega fatty acid imbalance with high-quality fish oil and by eliminating the seed oils that had been dominating his diet. We optimized his vitamin D with supplementation, getting his levels up to 62 ng/mL. We added zinc and magnesium, both essential cofactors for testosterone production that are commonly depleted in men under chronic stress.

As his terrain improved, his inflammatory markers dropped. His fasting insulin normalized. His energy continued to climb. And something remarkable happened: his body started producing testosterone again.

Four months after our first meeting, we repeated his labs. His testosterone had risen from 289 to 486 ng/dL - a 68% increase without any hormone replacement.[9] His free testosterone, the portion actually available for use, had increased even more dramatically. His SHBG (sex hormone binding globulin) had normalized, meaning more of his testosterone was bioavailable. His inflammatory markers were now in the optimal range. His fasting insulin had dropped from 18 to 6.

More importantly, he felt better than he had in years. His energy was strong and stable throughout the day, without the afternoon crashes he had grown accustomed to. His mood had improved - his wife commented that he seemed like himself again for the first time in years. His workouts produced results; he was building muscle and losing fat in ways that had seemed impossible before. His focus was sharper. His sleep was deeper. Even his libido had returned.

"If I had just taken the testosterone," Robert told me on that four-month visit, "I would still be eating garbage, still not sleeping, still inflamed. I might have felt a little better for a while, but everything underneath would have kept getting worse. Instead, I actually fixed the problem. And honestly, I feel better now than I would have on testosterone replacement, because everything is working the way it should."

The Bidirectional Relationship

There is one more piece of this puzzle that is important to understand: the relationship between terrain and hormones goes both ways. A dysfunctional terrain causes hormone imbalances, but hormone imbalances also damage the terrain.[37]

Low testosterone, for example, leads to increased body fat - especially visceral fat around the organs. This fat tissue is not just storage; it is metabolically active, producing inflammatory cytokines and contributing to insulin resistance. Low testosterone worsens the very terrain dysfunction that caused testosterone to drop in the first place.

Low thyroid function slows metabolism, which impairs detoxification. Toxins accumulate, further damaging mitochondria and worsening thyroid function. Estrogen dominance impairs liver function, and impaired liver function leads to poor estrogen clearance, worsening the dominance. Each imbalance feeds back on itself, creating a downward spiral that can be difficult to escape.

This is why early intervention matters. The longer terrain dysfunction persists, the more entrenched these feedback loops become. Robert caught his problem early, after just a few years of decline. Someone who has been in this downward spiral for decades may need more time and more intensive support to restore function. But restoration is almost always possible when you address the terrain rather than just replacing hormones.

Understanding how terrain dysfunction leads to hormone imbalance is crucial. But there is another piece of the puzzle that explains why some people can have normal - or even high - hormone levels on lab tests and still feel terrible. In the next chapter, we will explore the drainage problem - what happens when hormones cannot be properly delivered to tissues, processed by the liver, and cleared from the body.

Key Takeaways

- Hormone imbalances do not happen randomly - they are the body's intelligent response to dysfunctional terrain.
- The MILA axis - mitochondria, immune, and lymphatic - forms the foundation of terrain health.
- Mitochondrial dysfunction is at the root, but treatment must start with lymphatics and work backward.
- Terrain and hormones have a bidirectional relationship - each affects the other in a cycle that can spiral up or down.
- Restoring terrain can allow the body to resume normal hormone production without replacement therapy.

Chapter 3

When Hormones Can't Be Cleared

When Hormones Can't Be Cleared

Catherine was 44 years old and convinced something was seriously wrong with her hormones. She sat in my office holding a stack of lab results, pointing at the numbers with frustration.

"Look at this," she said. "My estrogen is actually on the higher end of normal. But I have every symptom of hormone imbalance you can imagine. My periods are heavy and painful - I go through a super tampon every hour on my worst days. My breasts are so tender before my period that I can barely hug my kids. I've gained fifteen pounds in the past year, all in my hips and thighs. I'm constantly bloated. My mood is all over the place. I cry at commercials. I snap at my husband for no reason."

Catherine was a veterinarian who had built a successful practice over two decades. She was used to solving diagnostic puzzles. But her own body had become a mystery she could not crack.

"My doctor said my hormones are fine - actually, she said my estrogen might even be a little high. She offered me birth control pills to regulate my cycle and an antidepressant for my mood. But that doesn't make sense to me. If my estrogen is high, why do I feel so terrible? And why would the solution be to add more hormones?"

Catherine had stumbled onto one of the most misunderstood aspects of hormone health. Her problem was not how much hormone her body was making. Her problem was that her body could not process, deliver, and clear those hormones properly. She was experiencing what happens when the drainage system fails.

The Two Ways Hormones Fail

When most people think about hormone problems, they think about deficiency. Not enough thyroid hormone. Not enough testosterone. Not enough estrogen. The solution seems obvious: measure what is low and replace it. But this simple model misses two other ways that hormones can fail to do their job.

The first is receptor dysfunction. Even when hormones are present in adequate amounts, cells may not be able to receive their messages. Inflammation, nutrient deficiencies, and fatty acid imbalances can all damage or block hormone receptors. You can have plenty of hormone circulating in your blood, but if your cells cannot hear the signal, you will have all the symptoms of deficiency. We will explore this problem in depth in the next chapter.[38]

The second - and often overlooked - problem is drainage failure. Hormones do not just need to be made and received.

They also need to be delivered to tissues, used, and then cleared from the body. When the systems responsible for hormone transport and clearance become congested, hormones and their breakdown products can build up in ways that cause serious problems.

This is the piece that most doctors miss entirely. They measure hormone levels in the blood and assume that tells the whole story. But blood levels do not tell you whether hormones are reaching tissues. They do not tell you whether hormones are being properly processed. And they do not tell you whether hormone breakdown products are being cleared - or accumulating in ways that cause harm.

The Lymphatic System: Your Body's Drainage Network

To understand drainage problems, you need to understand the lymphatic system. This network of vessels and nodes runs throughout your entire body, parallel to your blood vessels. It carries a clear fluid called lymph that bathes your tissues, delivers nutrients, removes waste products, and transports immune cells.[33]

Unlike your blood, which is pumped by your heart, lymph has no central pump. It relies on muscle movement, breathing, and the gentle contractions of the lymph vessels themselves to keep flowing.[39] This means that when you are sedentary, dehydrated, or chronically stressed, lymphatic flow slows dramatically. Waste products accumulate. Fluid builds up in tissues. And critically for our purposes, hormone breakdown products that should be cleared begin to back up.

The lymphatic system also plays a crucial role in getting hormones to their target tissues. Hormones released into the bloodstream must eventually reach the interstitial fluid - the fluid between cells - where they can interact with cell receptors. The lymphatic system helps maintain the proper flow and composition of this interstitial fluid.[40] When lymphatic flow is sluggish, this fluid becomes congested, and hormones may not reach their targets efficiently.

Think of it like a highway system. The blood vessels are the main highways bringing hormones from the glands where they are made. The lymphatic system is the network of local roads that distributes hormones to neighborhoods and also handles waste removal. When the local roads are jammed, it does not matter how much traffic is flowing on the highway - nothing is getting where it needs to go, and the garbage is piling up.

The Liver: Where Hormones Go to Be Processed

The liver is your body's primary hormone processing plant. After hormones have done their job, they travel to the liver to be broken down and prepared for elimination. This applies to all hormones - estrogen, testosterone, cortisol, thyroid hormones, and more. Each must be processed through the liver before it can be safely removed from your body. When the liver is overburdened, hormone clearance slows down across the board.[41]

Your liver breaks down hormones in two steps. In the first step, hormones are converted into breakdown products. Some of these breakdown products are harmless and easy for your body to eliminate. Others are more problematic - they can be more potent than the original hormone and harder for your body to clear.[41] Which type your body makes depends on your nutrition, your toxic burden, and how well your liver is functioning.

In the second step, your liver packages these breakdown products so they can be eliminated through your bile and urine. Think of it like putting garbage in a bag and tying it closed so it can go out with the trash.[42] If step one runs too fast or step two runs too slow, these breakdown products build up instead of being cleared. Either way, the result is the same: *hormone waste accumulates in your body instead of leaving.*

Why does it matter if these breakdown products accumulate? Because many of them are still active - some are even more potent than the original hormone. When they build up in your tissues, they keep stimulating your cells even after the original hormone has done its job. It is like a guest who will not leave the party. Your body senses all this hormone activity and may respond by reducing production of new hormones, throwing your levels off. Some of these breakdown products can also block hormone receptors, sitting in the lock without turning it, so real hormones cannot get their messages through. Others cause inflammation and can even damage cells over time. This is why proper hormone clearance is just as important as proper hormone production - and why you can have symptoms of hormone excess and hormone deficiency at the same time.

The liver does not work in isolation. It depends on adequate nutrients - B vitamins, magnesium, amino acids - to run these processing steps. It depends on healthy bile flow to eliminate the packaged waste. And it is intimately connected to the lymphatic system through the gut, where lymphatic vessels transport fats and fat-soluble compounds from the intestines to the liver for processing.

The Gut-Hormone Connection

Your gut bacteria play a surprising role in hormone balance - one that most people have never heard of.[43] After your liver packages up used hormones for removal, it sends them to your gut to be eliminated in your stool. But what happens next depends on the bacteria living in your intestines.

In a healthy gut with balanced bacteria, the packaged hormones leave your body as intended. But certain types of bacteria can unpackage those hormones, freeing them to be reabsorbed back into your bloodstream instead of being eliminated.[44] Think of it like a package you put out for the garbage truck. If someone opens the package before the truck arrives and brings the contents back inside, you never actually get rid of it. That is what happens with hormones when gut bacteria are out of balance.

Constipation makes this worse because it gives bacteria more time to work on the hormones before they leave your body. This is why gut health matters so much for hormone balance, and why the R.E.S.T.O.R.E. MILA protocol addresses the gut early in the healing process.

Catherine's Real Problem

When I evaluated Catherine's full picture, the drainage problem became clear. Her estrogen levels were not the issue. Her ability to process and clear estrogen was.

She had all the signs of lymphatic congestion. She was sedentary - running a busy veterinary practice meant long days on her feet but little actual movement or exercise. She drank coffee all day and very little water. She had chronic puffiness, especially in her face and around her ankles. Her sinuses were perpetually congested. She had tender, swollen lymph nodes that she had attributed to recurrent minor infections.

Her liver was burdened. She had a glass or two of wine most nights to unwind from the stress of work. She ate out frequently, consuming seed oils and processed foods without realizing it. Her diet was high in sugar and low in the cruciferous vegetables that support healthy hormone processing.[45] She took ibuprofen regularly for headaches - a medication that adds to liver burden.

Her gut was compromised. She had been on multiple courses of antibiotics over the years. She experienced bloating after meals and irregular bowel movements - sometimes constipated, sometimes loose. Stool testing revealed an overgrowth of bacteria associated with hormone recirculation.

We ran a specialized test that looked not just at her estrogen levels but at how her body was processing estrogen. The results were telling. Her body was producing far more of the problematic breakdown products than the protective ones - the exact pattern we see when the liver is overburdened and the drainage pathways are sluggish.[45] And her overall levels of these breakdown products were elevated, indicating that hormone waste was building up in her system instead of being cleared.

Catherine did not have an estrogen production problem. She had an estrogen clearance problem. Her body was making a normal amount of estrogen, but that estrogen was being processed through harmful pathways, building up as problematic breakdown products, and recirculating instead of being eliminated. No wonder she felt terrible despite normal blood levels.

Why Adding Hormones to a Clogged System Makes Things Worse

Catherine's doctor had suggested birth control pills to regulate her cycle. This is a common recommendation but think about what it actually means for someone with drainage problems. Birth control pills add synthetic hormones to a system that is already unable to clear the hormones it has.

It is like pouring more water into a sink that is already backing up because the drain is clogged. The water level rises higher. The overflow gets worse. The problem is not too little water - it is that the water cannot get out, adding more only makes things worse.

This is why hormone replacement so often fails or causes new problems. If the underlying drainage dysfunction is not addressed, adding more hormones - whether through pills, patches, pellets, or creams - just increases the burden on an already overwhelmed system. The liver has to process more. The lymphatics have to move more. The gut has to clear more. Eventually, symptoms get worse instead of better.[46]

The same principle applies to every hormone, not just estrogen. Testosterone that cannot be cleared can convert to estrogen and other breakdown products in excess. Thyroid hormone that cannot reach tissues, or be processed properly, builds up or converts to reverse T3. Cortisol that cannot be cleared continues to circulate, perpetuating the stress response. In every case, the answer is not more hormone - it is better drainage.

Opening the Drains

For Catherine, the solution was not to manipulate her hormone levels. It was to restore her body's ability to process and clear hormones properly. This meant addressing lymphatics, liver, and gut simultaneously.

We started with the lymphatic system. She began daily movement - not intense exercise, but consistent walking and gentle rebounding on a mini trampoline to stimulate lymphatic flow. She learned dry brushing, a technique that manually stimulates lymphatic drainage through the skin. She started deep breathing exercises, since the movement of the diaphragm is one of the primary pumps for lymphatic circulation. And she dramatically increased her water intake while reducing coffee and alcohol.

We supported her liver. She eliminated the Toxic Nine - sugar, wheat and gluten, corn, soy, dairy, peanuts, seed oils, alcohol, and chemical additives - reducing the burden on her liver's processing pathways. She added cruciferous vegetables daily to support healthy hormone processing. We supplemented DIM and calcium-d-glucarate to support both steps of liver processing.[47] She stopped the daily ibuprofen and addressed the root cause of her headaches, which turned out to be related to her lymphatic congestion.

We healed her gut. We used targeted probiotics to restore healthy bacterial balance. We addressed the bacterial overgrowth with antimicrobial herbs. We improved her bowel regularity with fiber, magnesium, and adequate hydration - ensuring that hormones packaged for elimination actually left her body promptly instead of sitting in the colon waiting to be recycled.

Catherine's Transformation

The changes came gradually, but they were unmistakable. Within the first month, Catherine's puffiness began to resolve. Her face looked less swollen in the mornings. Her rings fit more easily. The chronic sinus congestion that had plagued her for years started to clear.

By six weeks, her premenstrual symptoms had noticeably improved. The breast tenderness was dramatically reduced. The mood swings were less intense. She reported feeling more emotionally stable throughout her cycle.

By three months, her periods had transformed. The heavy bleeding had reduced significantly - she was no longer going through a tampon every hour. The painful cramping had diminished. Her cycle had become more regular. The weight that had accumulated in her hips and thighs began to shift.

We repeated her hormone processing test at the four-month mark. The pattern had reversed - she was now producing more of the protective breakdown products than the problematic ones. Her overall levels of these breakdown products had dropped significantly, indicating that hormones were now being cleared properly instead of accumulating.[45]

"My estrogen level on the regular blood test is actually a little lower now," Catherine told me at her four-month follow-up. "But I feel so much better. How is that possible?"

The answer was simple: her hormones were finally flowing properly. They were being delivered to tissues, used, processed through healthy pathways, and cleared. The traffic jam had been resolved. The drainage was working. Her body no longer needed to maintain a backup of hormones in her blood because the whole system was moving efficiently.

"What would have happened if I had just taken the birth control pills?" she asked.

"At best, you might have had some symptom relief while masking the underlying problem," I said. "At worst, you would have added more hormones to a system that couldn't clear them, potentially making the hormone imbalance worse over time. Either way, you would not have fixed anything - and the lymphatic congestion, liver burden, and gut dysfunction would have continued to cause problems, whether in your hormones or somewhere else."

The Receptor-Drainage Connection

Receptor dysfunction and drainage dysfunction are not separate problems. They are connected, and they often occur together.

When lymphatic flow is sluggish, inflammation increases - and inflammation damages receptors. When the liver is burdened, it produces inflammatory signals that affect receptor sensitivity throughout the body. When hormone breakdown products accumulate, they can compete with active hormones for receptor binding, blocking the signals that should be getting through.

This is why addressing drainage is often the first step in restoring hormone function - and why it is the foundation of the Eliminate phase in the R.E.S.T.O.R.E. MILA protocol. Until the drainage pathways are open and flowing, adding hormones or trying to sensitize receptors is likely to fail. You have to be able to clear waste before you can process new inputs efficiently.

This is also why the MILA axis lists the lymphatic system as one of its three pillars. Mitochondria produce the energy hormones need. The immune system affects inflammation and receptor function. And the lymphatic system determines whether hormones can flow freely through the body - reaching their targets, doing their jobs, and being cleared when their work is done. All three must be functioning for hormones to work properly.

Catherine's story shows what happens when hormones cannot be cleared. But there is another layer to hormone dysfunction that we have not yet explored - what happens when cells cannot receive hormone signals even when drainage is working. In the next chapter, we will look at receptor dysfunction and why some people need ever-increasing doses of hormones just to feel the same effect.

Key Takeaways

- Hormones can fail in three ways: deficiency (not enough made), resistance (receptors cannot respond), or congestion (cannot be delivered or cleared).
- The lymphatic system is essential for hormone delivery and clearance - when it becomes congested, hormones and their breakdown products build up.
- The liver processes all hormones, and when overburdened, breakdown products accumulate - causing symptoms of both hormone excess and deficiency at the same time.
- Adding hormones to a clogged system makes things worse - like pouring water into a sink with a clogged drain.
- Opening drainage pathways through lymphatic support, liver care, and gut healing often resolves hormone symptoms without any hormone manipulation.

Chapter 4

When Cells Can't Listen

When Cells Can't Listen

Angela was 45 years old and had been on hormone replacement therapy for three years. What had started as a solution had become a source of constant frustration.

"When I first started the hormones, I felt amazing," she told me. "It was like someone had turned the lights back on. My energy came back. My mood stabilized. My brain fog cleared. I thought I had found the answer."

Angela was a high school guidance counselor who prided herself on helping teenagers navigate difficult transitions. Now she was struggling to navigate her own. She had entered perimenopause at 42, and her doctor had started her on bioidentical hormone replacement - estrogen and progesterone - to manage her symptoms.

"The first year was great," she continued. "But then the symptoms started creeping back. The hot flashes returned. The sleep problems came back. My doctor increased my dose, and I felt better again - for a while. Then the same thing happened. More symptoms, higher dose. Better for a few months, then worse again."

She pulled out a piece of paper with her hormone history written on it.

"Look at this. I started on 0.5 mg of estradiol. Now I'm on 2 mg - four times my starting dose. And I still don't feel as good as I did that first year on the lower dose. My doctor says my levels look great on paper. But I feel terrible. How is that possible?"

Angela had stumbled onto one of the most overlooked problems in hormone therapy: receptor dysfunction. Her body was receiving plenty of hormones. But her cells had stopped listening.

The Phone That Stopped Ringing

To understand what was happening to Angela, think of hormones like phone calls and receptors like the phones that receive them. When a hormone reaches a cell, it needs to deliver a message. The receptor is what allows that message to get through.[48]

In a healthy system, the hormone dials the number, the receptor picks up, and communication happens. The cell gets the message and responds appropriately. But what happens when the phone is broken? What if the ringer is turned off? What if there is so much static on the line that the message cannot get through?

The caller - the hormone - is doing its job. The call is being made. But no communication is actually happening. You can shout louder into a broken phone, but it will not help. The problem is not the volume of the call. The problem is the phone itself.

This is exactly what happens with hormone receptor dysfunction. The hormones are present - sometimes in abundance - but the cells cannot receive their messages.[49] You can have all the symptoms of hormone deficiency even when blood tests show your hormone levels are perfectly normal or even high.

What Damages Hormone Receptors

Several things can impair your cells' ability to receive hormone signals. Understanding these helps explain why hormone replacement so often fails - and what actually needs to happen for hormones to work properly.

Chronic inflammation is one of the biggest culprits. When your body is in a constant state of low-grade inflammation, inflammatory signals interfere with hormone receptors throughout your body.[50] The receptors become less sensitive, like a phone with the volume turned down. This is well-documented with insulin - chronic inflammation is a major driver of insulin resistance, where cells stop responding to insulin even when plenty is present. But the same thing happens with estrogen receptors, thyroid receptors, and virtually every other type.

Cell membrane health also matters enormously. Many hormone receptors are embedded in the outer membrane of cells

- the wall that surrounds each cell. These membranes are made largely of fats. When the types of fats in your diet are out of balance - too many omega-6 fats from seed oils, not enough omega-3 fats from fish and other sources - cell membranes become stiff and rigid.[51] Receptors embedded in these rigid membranes cannot move and flex the way they need to. They cannot properly receive hormone signals.

Nutrient deficiencies play a role as well. Receptors are made of proteins and making them requires adequate building blocks from your diet. Many receptors also need specific vitamins and minerals to function properly. Zinc, for example, is essential for thyroid hormone receptors to work correctly.[18] Vitamin D is needed for its own receptors to be properly expressed. When these nutrients are lacking, receptors malfunction.

Environmental toxins can damage receptors directly. Many chemicals in our environment are classified as endocrine disruptors precisely because they interfere with hormone receptors.[52] Some toxins mimic hormones and bind to receptors themselves, blocking the real hormones from getting through. Others damage receptors or change how many receptors cells produce.

The Downregulation Trap

There is one more cause of receptor dysfunction that is particularly relevant for people on hormone replacement therapy: downregulation. This is what was happening to Angela, and it explains why she needed ever-increasing doses to feel the same effect.

When cells are constantly exposed to high levels of a hormone, they protect themselves by becoming less sensitive. They do this in two ways: they reduce the number of receptors on their surface, and they make the remaining receptors less responsive.[53] This is the body's way of protecting itself from overstimulation. It is a normal, intelligent adaptation.

The problem is that this creates a vicious cycle with hormone replacement. You start taking hormones and feel better because your cells are responding to the new signals. But over time, your cells adapt to higher hormone levels by reducing their receptors. Now you need more hormones to get the same effect. So, you increase the dose. You feel better for a while. Then your cells adapt again. You need even more. The cycle continues.

This is why so many people on hormone replacement describe the same pattern Angela experienced: initial improvement, followed by gradual return of symptoms, followed by dose increases, followed by brief improvement, followed by more symptoms. They are chasing a moving target. The more hormones they add, the more their receptors down-regulate, the more hormones they need.

Eventually, many people find themselves on extremely high doses of hormones and still feeling terrible. Their blood tests show plenty of hormone. But their cells have turned down the volume so far that the message is barely getting through.

The Reverse T3 Problem: A Special Case

There is a specific type of receptor blocking that deserves special attention because it affects so many people: the reverse T3 problem with thyroid hormones.

Your thyroid primarily produces a hormone called T4, which is a storage form. T4 must be converted to T3 to become active - T3 is what actually delivers messages to your cells. But there is another option: T4 can also be converted to something called reverse T3.[1]

Reverse T3 is like a broken key. It fits into the same receptors as regular T3, but it does not turn the lock. When reverse T3 is sitting in a receptor, real T3 cannot get in. The receptor is occupied but no message is being delivered. You can have plenty of T3 in your blood, but if reverse T3 is blocking the receptors, your cells are not getting the signal.

What causes the body to make more reverse T3? Stress, inflammation, and chronic illness.[3] When the body is under threat, it converts more T4 to reverse T3 as a way of slowing down metabolism and conserving resources. This is an intelligent survival mechanism. But in our modern world of chronic stress and ongoing inflammation, many people are stuck in this mode. They make plenty of thyroid hormone, but too much of it is being converted to the inactive reverse form that blocks receptors.

This is why so many people have all the symptoms of low thyroid function - fatigue, weight gain, brain fog, feeling cold - despite normal-looking thyroid labs. The standard tests do not measure reverse T3. They do not tell you whether the hormone that is present is actually getting into cells and doing its job.

Angela's Real Problem

When I evaluated Angela comprehensively, the receptor problem became clear. Her hormones were not the issue. Her cells' ability to respond to those hormones was.

Her inflammatory markers were elevated. Her C-reactive protein, a general marker of inflammation, was high. She had been eating what she thought was a healthy diet, but it was heavy in seed oils and processed foods that promote inflammation. Her omega-6 to omega-3 ratio was 18 to 1 - far from the ideal of 2 to 1 or less.

Her gut was inflamed. She had chronic bloating and irregular bowel movements. Testing revealed intestinal permeability - what is sometimes called leaky gut - which was allowing inflammatory proteins to enter her bloodstream and trigger immune responses throughout her body.[55]

Her nutrient status was poor, despite eating a reasonable diet. Her vitamin D was low at 26 ng/mL. Her zinc was at the bottom of the normal range. Her magnesium was depleted - not surprising, given the stress she was under. All of these nutrients are essential for proper receptor function.

And her thyroid, though not the primary hormone she was supplementing, showed the reverse T3 pattern. Her T3 levels looked adequate, but her reverse T3 was elevated, suggesting that even her thyroid hormones were being blocked at the receptor level. Her whole system was in a state of hormone resistance.

On top of all this, she had been on escalating doses of hormone replacement for three years. Her receptors had down-regulated in response to the chronically high hormone levels. She was caught in the trap - needing more and more hormones to overcome receptors that were becoming less and less responsive.

Why More Hormone Was Not the Answer

Angela's previous doctors had responded to her complaints the only way they knew how: by increasing her hormone doses. When she felt worse, they gave her more. This is the standard approach in conventional hormone replacement - treating the symptoms by adjusting the numbers.

But think about what this approach actually does. If the problem is that cells cannot hear hormone signals, adding louder signals does not fix the underlying issue. It is like turning up the volume on a radio with broken speakers. More volume does not repair the speakers. Eventually, you max out the volume and still cannot hear anything clearly.

Worse, adding more hormones when receptors are already down-regulated can trigger further down-regulation. The cells, already overwhelmed, turn down their sensitivity even more.

You end up needing ever-higher doses while getting ever-diminishing returns. This is not a path to health. It is a path to hormone dependency with progressively less benefit.

The real solution is not more hormones. The real solution is fixing the receptors so that whatever hormones are present - whether your own or from replacement - can actually do their job.

Restoring Receptor Function

For Angela, the goal was not to add more hormones. It was to restore her cells' ability to respond to the hormones she already had. This meant addressing the inflammation, nutrient deficiencies, and terrain dysfunction that were impairing her receptors.

We started with diet. She eliminated the Toxic Nine - sugar, wheat and gluten, corn, soy, dairy, peanuts, seed oils, alcohol, and chemical additives. The seed oils were particularly important because they were driving her omega fatty acid imbalance and contributing to rigid, dysfunctional cell membranes. We added high-quality fish oil to improve her omega-3 status.

We healed her gut. We addressed the intestinal permeability with targeted nutrients - glutamine, zinc carnosine, and collagen. We rebalanced her gut bacteria with specific probiotics. As her gut healed, the inflammatory proteins that had been leaking into her bloodstream decreased, and her systemic inflammation began to resolve.

More importantly, we began a slow, careful reduction in her hormone doses. This was not about stopping her hormones abruptly - that would have caused severe symptoms. It was about gradually reducing the hormone load to allow her receptors to resensitize. As her terrain improved and her inflammation decreased, her cells became better able to respond to lower doses.

Angela's Transformation

The process was not instant, receptor healing takes time. But the changes, when they came, were profound.

Within six weeks, Angela's inflammatory markers had begun to drop and her bloating had resolved. She was sleeping better - not perfectly, but better. And though we had actually reduced her estrogen dose slightly, she was not feeling worse. If anything, she was feeling a little better.

By three months, the transformation was becoming clear. Her C-reactive protein had normalized. Her omega fatty acid ratio had improved from 18 to 1 down to 6 to 1 - still not ideal, but dramatically better. Her energy was improving. Her hot flashes had decreased even though her estrogen dose was now half of what it had been when we started.

By six months, Angela was on a lower dose of hormones than she had been at any point in the past two years - and feeling better than she had felt in years. Her symptoms were well-controlled. Her sleep had normalized. Her mood was stable. Her thinking was clear.

"I don't understand it," she told me. "I'm on less hormone than ever, but I feel better than I did on the highest dose. How is that possible?"

"Because it was never about the amount of hormone," I explained. "It was about whether your cells could hear the message. When your receptors were damaged and down-regulated, even high doses couldn't get through. Now that we've fixed the underlying problems, lower doses work better than the high doses ever did. Your cells are finally listening."

Angela continued to maintain her terrain-supportive diet and lifestyle. Over the following year, we were able to reduce her hormones further. She did not come off them entirely - she was still in menopause and her ovaries were no longer producing significant hormones. But she stabilized on a low dose that kept her symptoms controlled without overwhelming her receptors. She had escaped the down-regulation trap.

Angela's story shows what happens when receptors cannot respond to hormones. But there is another layer to hormone dysfunction that involves the immune system itself. In the next chapter, we will explore what happens when your body produces antibodies against your own hormone-producing glands - and why these antibodies may not be the enemies we have been taught to believe they are.

Key Takeaways

- Hormone receptors are like phones - if they are damaged or turned off, it does not matter how many calls come in.
- Inflammation, poor cell membrane health, nutrient deficiencies, and toxins can all damage hormone receptors.
- Down-regulation is a trap - the more hormone you add, the less sensitive your receptors become, requiring ever-higher doses.
- Reverse T3 can block thyroid receptors, causing hypothyroid symptoms despite normal thyroid hormone levels.
- Fixing the terrain - reducing inflammation, improving cell membranes, correcting nutrients - allows receptors to heal so that lower hormone doses work better than high doses ever did.

Chapter 5

The Autoimmune Connection

When Your Body Attacks Its Own Hormones

Melissa was 38 years old when she received the diagnosis that changed how she thought about her body. After years of fatigue, weight gain, and feeling cold all the time, a doctor finally ran the right tests. Her thyroid peroxidase antibodies were elevated at 412 IU/mL - well above the normal range of less than 35. She had Hashimoto's thyroiditis.

"Your immune system is attacking your thyroid," her endocrinologist explained. "It's an autoimmune disease. There's no cure. Eventually your thyroid will be destroyed, and you'll need to be on thyroid medication for the rest of your life. We should start you on levothyroxine now to protect whatever thyroid function you have left."

Melissa left that appointment feeling devastated. Her body had turned against itself. Her immune system - the very thing designed to protect her - had become the enemy. She imagined little soldiers inside her, systematically dismantling her thyroid gland cell by cell. She went home and researched Hashimoto's, finding story after story of people whose thyroid function had progressively declined despite medication, whose antibody levels remained stubbornly high, who had resigned themselves to a lifetime of managing an incurable disease.

"I felt like my body had betrayed me," Melissa told me when she came to my office six months later. "Like I was at war with myself and there was nothing I could do but watch my thyroid get destroyed."

What Melissa did not know - what her endocrinologist had not explained - was that the story she had been told about thyroid antibodies was incomplete. Her immune system was not randomly attacking her thyroid. It was responding to something. And if we could figure out what that something was, we might be able to change the entire trajectory of her disease.

The Autoimmune Story We Have Been Told

The conventional understanding of autoimmune thyroid disease goes something like this: for reasons we do not fully understand, the immune system becomes confused and starts attacking the body's own tissues. In Hashimoto's thyroiditis, it attacks the thyroid gland. In Graves' disease, it overstimulates it. The immune system has made a mistake - it has identified itself as foreign and launched an inappropriate attack.[56]

This story frames the immune system as the villain. Antibodies are the weapons of destruction. Treatment focuses on suppressing symptoms (with thyroid hormone replacement) or suppressing the immune system itself (with immunosuppressive drugs in more severe cases). The underlying assumption is that the immune response is the problem.

But what if this story is wrong? What if the immune system is not making a mistake at all? What if the antibodies are not the cause of the disease, but the body's attempt to respond to an underlying problem?

A Different Way to Understand Antibodies

The immune system does not attack tissues randomly. It is exquisitely designed to distinguish self from non-self, and it has multiple fail-safes to prevent attacking the body's own cells.[57] When we see the immune system targeting a specific tissue, the question we should ask is: why? What is the immune system responding to?

In many cases of so-called autoimmune disease, the immune system is actually doing its job correctly. It is responding to a genuine threat - but the threat is not the tissue itself. The threat might be a pathogen that has taken up residence in that tissue. It might be toxins that have accumulated there. It might be damaged cells that need to be cleared away. The immune system is not confused. It is trying to address a real problem.[58]

Consider what we know about the thyroid gland specifically. The thyroid concentrates iodine from the bloodstream - it is one of the few tissues in the body that actively accumulates this element. But the thyroid also concentrates other halogens that share chemical similarities with iodine: fluoride, bromide, and chlorine compounds.[59] These toxic halogens are everywhere in our modern environment - in our water supply, our food, our flame retardants, our medications. When they accumulate in the thyroid, they can damage thyroid cells and trigger an immune response.

The thyroid is also vulnerable to certain infections. Epstein-Barr virus, the virus that causes mononucleosis, has been strongly linked to Hashimoto's thyroiditis.[60] Other viruses and bacteria can also infect thyroid tissue. When the immune system detects these pathogens in the thyroid, it mounts a response - and that response can look like the immune system is attacking the thyroid itself.

Gut dysfunction plays a major role as well. When the intestinal barrier becomes permeable - a condition often called leaky gut - proteins can escape from the digestive tract into the bloodstream. Some of these proteins look similar to thyroid tissue proteins. The immune system, appropriately responding to these foreign proteins, can develop antibodies that cross-react with the thyroid.[61] This is called molecular mimicry, and it is one of the most well-documented mechanisms linking gut health to thyroid autoimmunity.

From this perspective, thyroid antibodies are not the disease. They are evidence that the immune system has detected a problem and is trying to respond. The antibodies are more like firefighters arriving at a burning building than arsonists setting the fire.

What the Research Actually Shows

This is not just theory. Research supports the idea that thyroid antibodies are a response to underlying problems, not a random malfunction of the immune system. The evidence comes from multiple directions, and it all points to the same conclusion: address the triggers, and the antibodies often decrease.

Studies have shown that eliminating gluten can significantly reduce thyroid antibody levels in people with Hashimoto's - even in people who do not have celiac disease.[61] In one study, patients who followed a strict gluten-free diet for six months showed a 40% reduction in thyroid antibodies compared to those who continued eating gluten. Why would removing a food protein affect thyroid antibodies? Because gluten can trigger intestinal permeability, allowing proteins into the bloodstream that cross-react with thyroid tissue. The gluten protein gliadin shares structural similarities with thyroid tissue proteins. When the immune system creates antibodies against gliadin, those same antibodies can mistakenly target the thyroid. Remove the trigger, reduce the antibodies.

Selenium supplementation has been shown to reduce thyroid antibodies in multiple studies.[62] A meta-analysis of randomized controlled trials found that selenium supplementation reduced TPO antibodies by an average of 40% over three to twelve months. Selenium is essential for the enzymes that protect the thyroid from oxidative damage - specifically, the glutathione peroxidases that neutralize hydrogen peroxide produced during thyroid hormone synthesis. When selenium is deficient, thyroid cells are more vulnerable to oxidative damage, and damaged cells trigger immune responses. Provide the nutrient, reduce the damage, reduce the antibodies.

Vitamin D deficiency has been strongly linked to thyroid autoimmunity.[63] Studies show that people with Hashimoto's have significantly lower vitamin D levels than healthy controls, and that lower vitamin D correlates with higher antibody levels. Vitamin D is not just a vitamin - it is a hormone that regulates immune function, helping to prevent the immune system from attacking the body's own tissues. When vitamin D is deficient, this regulatory function is impaired, and autoimmune responses become more likely. Supplementing vitamin D to optimal levels has been shown to reduce thyroid antibodies in some studies, though the effect is most pronounced when combined with other interventions.

Treating underlying infections has been shown to reduce or eliminate thyroid antibodies in some patients.[59] Epstein-Barr virus, in particular, has been found in thyroid tissue of people with Hashimoto's at much higher rates than in healthy controls. The virus appears to trigger an immune response that cross-reacts with thyroid proteins. Helicobacter pylori, the bacterium that causes stomach ulcers, has also been linked to thyroid autoimmunity - eradicating the infection has been shown to reduce thyroid antibodies in some patients. If the immune system was simply confused and attacking randomly, why would treating an infection change anything? Because the infection was the trigger the immune system was actually responding to.

The gut microbiome plays a crucial role that is only beginning to be understood.[3] Research shows that people with Hashimoto's have different gut bacteria profiles than healthy controls - specifically, they tend to have reduced diversity and an overgrowth of certain problematic species. When researchers have used probiotics to restore healthier gut bacteria, thyroid antibodies have decreased in some studies. The gut is where 70% of the immune system resides, and an unhealthy gut creates an unhealthy immune response.

Perhaps most tellingly, many people with elevated thyroid antibodies never develop thyroid dysfunction at all.[64] Studies following people with elevated antibodies over time find that only a portion - somewhere between 20% and 50% depending on the study - go on to develop hypothyroidism. If the antibodies themselves were directly destroying the thyroid, this would not make sense. But if the antibodies are a response to an underlying problem, it makes perfect sense - some people's immune systems manage to address the problem without significant collateral damage to the thyroid, while others experience more tissue destruction in the process. The difference likely lies in the severity and duration of the underlying triggers, and in individual variations in immune response.

Melissa's Real Problem

When I evaluated Melissa's full picture, the story behind her antibodies became clearer. Her immune system was not malfunctioning. It was responding to multiple legitimate triggers.

She had a history of mononucleosis in college - Epstein-Barr virus infection. Testing revealed that her Epstein-Barr antibodies were still elevated, suggesting the virus had reactivated or never fully gone dormant. This virus has a particular affinity for thyroid tissue and is strongly associated with Hashimoto's.

Her gut was compromised. She had been on multiple courses of antibiotics over the years for recurrent sinus infections. Stool testing revealed significant dysbiosis - an imbalance of gut bacteria - along with markers suggesting intestinal permeability. Her gut barrier was not intact, allowing proteins to leak into her bloodstream.

Her diet was heavy in gluten and dairy - two of the most common triggers for intestinal permeability and immune activation. She was also consuming significant amounts of soy, which contains compounds called goitrogens that can interfere with thyroid function and potentially trigger immune responses against thyroid tissue.

Her selenium level was low. Her vitamin D was deficient at 22 ng/mL. Both of these nutrients are critical for proper immune regulation and thyroid protection. Her omega fatty acid ratio was imbalanced at 16 to 1, promoting inflammation throughout her body.

She had significant toxic burden. Mineral analysis revealed elevated levels of mercury and arsenic. She drank unfiltered tap water, which in her area contained elevated fluoride - a halogen that competes with iodine in the thyroid and can trigger immune responses.

Looking at this picture, Melissa's thyroid antibodies made complete sense. Her immune system was not confused or malfunctioning. It was responding to viral infection, gut-derived proteins, toxic accumulation, and ongoing inflammatory triggers. The antibodies were not the problem - they were evidence that her body was trying to deal with multiple problems.

A Different Approach

Melissa's endocrinologist had focused on the thyroid itself - monitoring thyroid hormone levels and preparing to replace them when they inevitably declined. This approach accepts the antibodies as an unstoppable force and simply tries to manage the damage they cause.

We took a different approach. Instead of accepting the antibodies as inevitable, we asked what was triggering them - and then addressed those triggers.

Melissa eliminated the Toxic Nine - sugar, wheat and gluten, corn, soy, dairy, peanuts, seed oils, alcohol, and chemical additives. For her, gluten and soy were particularly important given their documented effects on thyroid autoimmunity. Within weeks, her chronic bloating resolved and her energy began improving.

We healed her gut. We used targeted antimicrobials to address the dysbiosis, specific probiotics to restore healthy bacteria, and gut-healing nutrients to repair her intestinal barrier. As her gut healed, the stream of inflammatory proteins entering her bloodstream slowed.

We addressed the Epstein-Barr virus with immune-supportive nutrients and specific antivirals. We supported her body's ability to keep the virus dormant rather than allowing it to continuously trigger immune activation.

We corrected her nutrient deficiencies. Selenium at 200 micrograms daily to protect her thyroid from oxidative damage. Vitamin D to optimal levels. Zinc for immune regulation. Omega-3 fatty acids to reduce inflammation and improve cell membrane function.

We reduced her toxic burden. She installed a water filter that removed fluoride and other contaminants. We supported her detoxification pathways with targeted nutrients. We identified and eliminated sources of mercury and arsenic exposure.

We did not suppress her immune system. We did not try to stop the antibodies directly. We simply removed the triggers that were causing her immune system to respond in the first place.

Melissa's Transformation

The changes were gradual but unmistakable. By three months, Melissa's energy had significantly improved. The brain fog that had plagued her was lifting. She was losing weight without trying - her body was finally able to function properly.

By six months, we repeated her labs. Her thyroid peroxidase antibodies had dropped from 412 to 187 - still elevated, but more than 50% lower than when she started. Her thyroid function, which had been borderline low, had actually improved. Her TSH had dropped from 4.8 to 2.3. Her free T3 and free T4 had both increased.

By one year, her antibodies had dropped to 64 - within striking distance of normal. Her thyroid function was solidly in the optimal range. She had never needed thyroid medication.

"My endocrinologist was shocked," Melissa told me. "She said she had never seen antibodies drop like that. She asked what I was doing, and when I explained, she said it must be a coincidence - that Hashimoto's doesn't work that way."

Melissa paused and shook her head.

"But it does work that way. The antibodies weren't the disease. They were my body's response to things that were actually wrong - the virus, the gut dysfunction, the toxins, the nutrient deficiencies. Once we fixed those things, my immune system didn't need to respond anymore. The firefighters left because the fire was out."

Beyond Thyroid: Antibodies Throughout the Hormone System

What applies to thyroid antibodies applies to hormone antibodies throughout the body. The same pattern - immune response to underlying triggers, rather than random autoimmune attack - can be seen in virtually every hormone-producing tissue. Understanding this opens up new possibilities for prevention and treatment that the conventional approach completely misses.

Ovarian antibodies are found in a significant percentage of women with premature ovarian failure - the early loss of ovarian function that leads to menopause before age 40. Conventional medicine treats this as an irreversible condition, offering only hormone replacement to manage the symptoms of early menopause. But the question that rarely gets asked is: why is the immune system targeting the ovaries in the first place?

Research has identified several potential triggers for ovarian autoimmunity. Viral infections, particularly mumps, have been linked to ovarian antibodies - the virus can infect ovarian tissue and trigger an immune response that persists long after the acute infection resolves. Environmental toxins that accumulate in fatty tissues, including the ovaries, can damage cells and trigger immune responses. Gut dysfunction and intestinal permeability can lead to the same molecular mimicry that affects the thyroid -

food proteins entering the bloodstream that cross-react with ovarian tissue.

Women with ovarian antibodies often have antibodies to other tissues as well - thyroid antibodies are particularly common. This suggests that the underlying problem is not specific to the ovaries but reflects a broader pattern of immune dysregulation driven by terrain dysfunction. Address the terrain, calm the immune system, and the attack on multiple tissues can potentially be reduced or halted.

Adrenal antibodies are found in Addison's disease, the autoimmune destruction of the adrenal glands that leads to cortisol deficiency. This is a serious condition that can be life-threatening if untreated, and once the adrenal glands are significantly damaged, cortisol replacement becomes necessary. But here too, the question of triggers is crucial - especially for people in the early stages, or those who have adrenal antibodies but have not yet developed full-blown Addison's disease.

The adrenal glands, like the thyroid, are vulnerable to certain infections. Tuberculosis was historically a common cause of adrenal destruction before antibiotics became available. Today, fungal infections and certain viruses can trigger adrenal autoimmunity. The adrenals are also sensitive to toxic burden - they concentrate certain heavy metals and are particularly vulnerable to oxidative stress. People with adrenal antibodies often show evidence of these underlying triggers when thoroughly evaluated.

Pancreatic beta cell antibodies are the hallmark of Type 1 diabetes, where the immune system destroys the insulin-producing cells of the pancreas. This has long been considered a purely genetic autoimmune disease with no known cause or prevention. But emerging research is challenging this view. Studies have found that certain viral infections - particularly enteroviruses - can trigger the autoimmune process in genetically susceptible individuals. Cow's milk protein introduced early in infancy has been linked to increased risk of beta cell antibodies in some studies, possibly through molecular mimicry.

Perhaps most intriguingly, vitamin D deficiency during pregnancy and early childhood has been associated with increased risk of Type 1 diabetes. Countries with less sunlight have higher rates of disease. Vitamin D supplementation in infancy appears to reduce risk. This suggests that immune dysregulation driven by nutrient deficiency may play a role even in this supposedly genetic condition.

The implications are profound. If we can identify people with early-stage antibodies before significant tissue destruction has occurred - and if we can identify and address their specific triggers - we may be able to prevent or slow the progression to full-blown disease. This is not yet standard practice in conventional medicine, where antibodies are typically only measured after symptoms have appeared and significant damage has already occurred. But it represents a fundamentally different approach: instead of waiting for disease and then managing damage, we identify risk early and address root causes.

In each case, the same questions apply: What is triggering the immune response? What infections, toxins, dietary factors, or terrain imbalances are causing the immune system to target these tissues? And what happens if we address those underlying triggers instead of simply managing the downstream damage?

The answer, in case after case, is that addressing the triggers can change the trajectory of the disease. Not always, and not completely in every case - some damage, once done, cannot be fully reversed. But the progression can often be halted. The antibodies can often be reduced. And the body's hormone-producing tissues can often be protected or even partially restored.

Understanding that antibodies are responses rather than causes changes how we approach hormone health. But there is one hormone that sits above all others in the hierarchy - one that, when dysfunctional, can throw every other hormone system into chaos. In the next chapter, we will explore insulin as the master regulator of metabolism, and why addressing insulin resistance is often the key to unlocking hormone balance throughout the body.

Key Takeaways

- Hormone antibodies are usually responses to underlying triggers, not random immune system malfunctions.
- Common triggers include viral infections, gut dysfunction, toxic exposures, nutrient deficiencies, and dietary proteins that cross-react with hormone tissues.

- Research shows that removing triggers - like gluten, infections, and toxins - can significantly reduce antibody levels.
- Treating antibodies as the enemy misses the point - they are more like firefighters responding to a fire than arsonists starting one.
- Addressing the underlying triggers through terrain restoration can halt disease progression and protect hormone-producing tissues.

Chapter 6

The Glucose Trap

Insulin: The Master Regulator

Gerald was 58 years old and had been fighting Type 2 diabetes for twelve years. What had started as slightly elevated blood sugar had progressed despite everything his doctors threw at it - first metformin, then a second medication, then a third. Now he was on insulin injections, and his doctor was talking about increasing the dose again.

"I don't understand it," Gerald told me at our first meeting, frustration evident in his voice. "I've done everything they asked. I take my medications. I try to watch what I eat. But my blood sugar keeps getting worse, not better. And I've gained forty pounds since I started the insulin. My doctor says that's normal - that insulin causes weight gain. But how is gaining weight supposed to help my diabetes?"

Gerald was a retired postal worker who had spent thirty years walking a mail route. He had always been active, always lean. The weight had crept on after retirement, and with it came the diabetes diagnosis. Now he felt trapped in a body he didn't recognize, dependent on medications that seemed to be making him worse, not better.

"The worst part," he continued, "is that I feel like I'm being punished for something I didn't do. Everyone acts like I gave myself diabetes by eating too much sugar. But I never had a sweet tooth. I ate the same way my whole life, and I was fine until I wasn't. What changed?"

What Gerald didn't know - what his doctors had never explained - was that his diabetes wasn't caused by eating too much sugar alone. Yes, sugar contributes to the problem, and reducing it is important. But diabetes is not primarily a disease of blood sugar - it is a disease of insulin resistance. Insulin resistance is itself a symptom of something deeper: terrain dysfunction that had been building for years before his blood sugar ever went up.

Why Insulin Sits at the Top of the Hormone Hierarchy

Throughout this book, we have discussed hormone imbalances as symptoms of terrain dysfunction. We have seen how the MILA axis - mitochondria, immune, and lymphatic - creates the foundation on which all hormone function depends. But among all the hormones in the body, insulin occupies a unique position. It is not just one hormone among many. It is the master regulator that influences every other hormone system.

Insulin's primary job is directing traffic for energy. When you eat, blood sugar rises. Insulin signals cells to take up that sugar and either use it immediately or store it for later. When insulin is working properly, this system keeps blood sugar in a narrow, healthy range while ensuring that cells have the fuel they need.

But insulin does far more than manage blood sugar. It influences virtually every metabolic process in the body. It determines whether you store fat or burn it. It affects protein synthesis and muscle building. It modulates inflammation throughout the body.[65] And critically for our purposes, it directly impacts every other hormone system - thyroid, adrenal, and reproductive hormones are all affected by insulin status.

When insulin function becomes impaired - a condition we call insulin resistance - the effects ripple throughout the entire endocrine system. High insulin levels suppress growth hormone. They increase cortisol. They convert testosterone to estrogen in men and drive testosterone overproduction in women. They impair thyroid hormone conversion.[66] A person with insulin resistance doesn't just have a blood sugar problem. They have a whole-body hormone problem.

This is why insulin resistance is found in the background of so many chronic conditions. Polycystic ovary syndrome, the most common hormonal disorder in women of reproductive age, is fundamentally driven by insulin resistance.[3] Many cases of low testosterone in men have insulin resistance as their root cause. Thyroid dysfunction often improves when insulin sensitivity is restored. The hormone imbalances that bring people to doctors' offices are frequently downstream effects of insulin dysfunction that no one thought to check.

Insulin Resistance: Protection Gone Wrong

To understand Gerald's condition, we need to understand what insulin resistance actually is - and what it isn't. Conventional medicine treats insulin resistance as though cells have simply become deaf to insulin signals for no particular reason. The solution, in this view, is to shout louder - give more insulin, add medications that force cells to respond, override the resistance by brute force.

But this view misses something crucial. Cells don't become resistant to insulin randomly. They become resistant because they are already overwhelmed.[3] Insulin resistance is not a malfunction. It is a protective mechanism - an intelligent cellular response to a situation where accepting more glucose would cause harm.

Think of it this way. Imagine a warehouse that receives deliveries of goods. When the warehouse has plenty of space and workers to process shipments, deliveries flow smoothly. The warehouse happily accepts everything that arrives. But what happens when the warehouse gets backed up? When previous shipments haven't been processed, when goods are piling up in the aisles, when workers are overwhelmed? The warehouse starts refusing new deliveries. It's not broken - it's protecting itself from collapse.

This is exactly what happens in insulin resistance. The "warehouse" is the cell. The "goods" are glucose. And the "workers" that process the glucose are the mitochondria. When mitochondria are functioning well, they efficiently convert glucose into ATP - the energy currency that powers cellular function. But when mitochondria are damaged, dysfunctional, or simply overwhelmed, glucose backs up. It can't be processed fast enough. And excess glucose inside cells is toxic - it damages proteins, produces harmful byproducts, and accelerates cellular aging.

Faced with this situation, the cell does something intelligent: it reduces its insulin receptors. It makes itself less sensitive to insulin's signal to take up more glucose. This is not a mistake or a malfunction. This is the cell protecting itself from glucose toxicity. The cell is saying, in effect, "I can't handle more fuel right now. Stop sending it."

Why Conventional Treatment Often Makes Things Worse

Once we understand insulin resistance as a protective response to cellular overwhelm, the problems with conventional diabetes treatment become painfully clear. Most conventional treatments don't address why cells are resisting glucose. They simply override the resistance, forcing glucose into cells that are already struggling to process it.

Consider the most common diabetes medications. Some drugs force the pancreas to produce more insulin, overwhelming cellular resistance through sheer volume. Others make cells more sensitive to insulin, essentially removing the protective barrier that cells had put up for good reason. Insulin injections bypass the body's regulatory mechanisms entirely, driving glucose into cells regardless of their capacity to handle it.[67]

The result? Blood sugar numbers may improve - at least initially. But the underlying problem gets worse, not better. Cells that were already overwhelmed become more overwhelmed. Mitochondria that were already struggling become more damaged. The metabolic dysfunction that caused the insulin resistance in the first place accelerates.

This explains why Type 2 diabetes is considered a "progressive" disease - why patients typically need more and more medication over time, why they often eventually end up on insulin, why complications continue to develop despite treatment.[68] The disease isn't progressing on its own. The treatment is driving progression by forcing glucose into cells that can't handle it, accelerating the mitochondrial damage that caused the problem in the first place.

Gerald's experience was a textbook example of this pattern. Each medication seemed to help initially, then stopped working. Each escalation bought temporary improvement followed by continued decline. And the insulin - supposedly the ultimate solution - was making him gain weight, which worsened his insulin resistance, which required higher doses, which caused more weight gain. He was caught in a vicious cycle that his treatment was driving, not solving.

The GLP-1 Medications: A Different Approach with Its Own Problems

In recent years, a new class of diabetes medications has emerged that works differently from traditional treatments. GLP-1 receptor agonists - including semaglutide (Ozempic, Wegovy) and tirzepatide (Mounjaro, Zepbound) - have taken the medical world by storm, initially for diabetes but increasingly for weight loss.[69]

These medications work by mimicking GLP-1, a hormone naturally produced in the gut after eating. GLP-1 signals the pancreas to release insulin in response to food, slows stomach emptying so you feel full longer, and acts on the brain to reduce appetite. The medications amplify these effects dramatically, leading to significant reductions in both blood sugar and body weight.

In some ways, this is a more intelligent approach than simply forcing glucose into cells. By reducing appetite and slowing digestion, these medications reduce the glucose load that cells have to deal with. People eat less, absorb sugar more slowly, and their overwhelmed cells get some relief.[70] The weight loss that typically accompanies these medications can also improve insulin sensitivity - less body fat means less inflammation and better metabolic function.

But there are significant problems with this approach that are only beginning to be understood. First, these medications don't fix the underlying terrain dysfunction - they just reduce the load on a dysfunctional system.[6] The mitochondria are still damaged. The inflammatory processes are still active. The MILA axis is still compromised. When the medication is stopped - and studies show that the vast majority of people regain weight after stopping - the underlying dysfunction reasserts itself.

Second, there are concerning effects on body composition. The weight lost on GLP-1 medications isn't just fat - a significant portion is muscle mass.[64] Some studies suggest that up to 40% of weight loss may be lean tissue rather than fat. This matters because muscle is metabolically active - it's where much of our glucose is used. Losing muscle mass may actually worsen insulin resistance in the long run, even as the scale shows improvement.

Third, and perhaps most importantly, these medications create a new form of dependency. The appetite suppression and metabolic effects only last as long as you take the medication. Stop the drug, and appetite returns - often with a vengeance. The body, having adapted to artificially suppressed hunger signals, may overshoot in the other direction.[71] Many people find themselves unable to stop the medication without rapid weight regain, committing to what may be lifelong treatment with drugs whose long-term effects are not yet fully understood.

Gerald's Real Problem

When I evaluated Gerald comprehensively, the picture that emerged was quite different from simple "diabetes." Yes, his blood sugar was poorly controlled. Yes, he met all the diagnostic criteria for Type 2 diabetes. But these were downstream effects of a much broader pattern of terrain dysfunction.

His mitochondrial function was severely compromised. An organic acids test revealed multiple markers of mitochondrial dysfunction - his cells were struggling to produce energy efficiently, exactly the pattern that drives insulin resistance. Years of a diet high in seed oils and processed foods had damaged the very organelles that needed to process glucose.

His inflammation was chronic and significant. His C-reactive protein was elevated. His fasting insulin was high - not normal, but high, indicating that his pancreas was working overtime trying to overcome his cells' resistance. This chronic hyperinsulinemia was itself inflammatory, creating a vicious cycle.[65]

His omega fatty acid ratio was dramatically imbalanced at 19 to 1 - almost ten times worse than optimal. This meant his cell membranes, including the membranes where insulin receptors sit, were rigid and dysfunctional. Insulin was binding to receptors that couldn't transduce the signal properly.

His gut was a disaster. Stool testing revealed severe dysbiosis, an overgrowth of bacteria that produce endotoxins - inflammatory molecules that directly impair insulin signaling. He had been on multiple rounds of antibiotics over the years for various infections, each one further disrupting his gut ecosystem.[64]

His vitamin D was deficient at 18 ng/mL - far below the optimal range of 50-80. Vitamin D deficiency is independently associated with insulin resistance. His magnesium was depleted, another factor that impairs insulin sensitivity. His B vitamins, critical for mitochondrial function, were suboptimal.

Looking at this picture, Gerald's diabetes made complete sense - not as a primary disease, but as a downstream consequence of years of accumulated terrain dysfunction. His cells weren't resisting insulin because they were broken. They were resisting insulin because they were overwhelmed, inflamed, and unable to process the glucose they were already forced to accept.

A Different Path

Gerald's conventional doctors had focused entirely on his blood sugar numbers. Every intervention was designed to force those numbers down, regardless of the cost to his underlying health. Our approach was fundamentally different: instead of overriding his cells' protective responses, we asked why they were protecting themselves in the first place - and addressed those root causes.

Gerald eliminated the Toxic Nine - sugar, wheat and gluten, corn, soy, dairy, peanuts, seed oils, alcohol, and chemical additives. For him, the seed oils were particularly important. He had been cooking everything in "heart-healthy" vegetable oils for decades, not realizing that these oils were destroying his mitochondrial membranes and driving insulin resistance. We replaced them with olive oil, avocado oil, and beef tallow.

We dramatically restructured his eating pattern. Instead of the frequent small meals he had been told to eat to "keep blood sugar stable," we moved him toward a time-restricted eating window.[72] This gave his insulin levels time to come down between meals - something that never happened when he was eating every few hours. The periods of low insulin allowed his cells to finally process the glucose backlog and begin to heal.

We supported his mitochondria directly with targeted nutrients - CoQ10, which is essential for mitochondrial energy production; alpha-lipoic acid, which improves both mitochondrial function and insulin sensitivity; and B vitamins to support the enzymatic machinery of energy production.

We healed his gut with antimicrobials to reduce the bacterial overgrowth, probiotics to restore healthy flora, and gut-healing nutrients to repair his intestinal barrier. As his gut healed, the inflammatory endotoxins that had been impairing his insulin signaling decreased.

We corrected his fatty acid imbalance with high-quality fish oil while eliminating the seed oils that were poisoning his cell membranes. Over time, his cell membranes became more fluid, more flexible, and more responsive to insulin signals.

We optimized his vitamin D, magnesium, and other nutrients that support insulin sensitivity. None of these alone would have fixed his diabetes. But together, they addressed the terrain dysfunction that had been driving his insulin resistance for years.

Gerald's Transformation

The changes didn't happen overnight. Reversing twelve years of metabolic dysfunction takes time. But the trajectory was unmistakable from early on.

Within the first month, Gerald's blood sugar variability improved dramatically. The wild swings that had plagued him - high after meals, crashing a few hours later - smoothed out. His continuous glucose monitor showed more time in range without us changing his medications at all.

By three months, we had been able to reduce his insulin dose. His hemoglobin A1c, which had been 8.2 despite maximum medical therapy, dropped to 7.1. His fasting blood sugar, once routinely in the 180s, was now averaging 130. And perhaps most remarkably, he had lost twenty pounds - not by forcing himself to eat less, but because his appetite had naturally normalized as his hormones came into balance.

By six months, Gerald was off insulin entirely. His A1c had dropped to 6.4 - still technically in the diabetic range, but barely. His fasting glucose was consistently under 110. His inflammatory markers had normalized. His omega fatty acid ratio had improved to 5 to 1 - still not perfect, but dramatically better.

He had lost thirty-five pounds in total and felt better than he had in decades.

"I finally understand what went wrong," Gerald told me on his six-month visit. "It wasn't just about sugar - though cutting that helped. It was that everything in my diet - the vegetable oils, the processed foods, the constant snacking - was poisoning my cells until they couldn't handle fuel anymore. The diabetes was my body trying to protect itself, and the insulin injections were just overriding that protection while making the underlying problem worse."

At one year, Gerald's A1c was 5.9 - technically no longer diabetic by laboratory standards. He had maintained his weight loss. He was able to discontinue all diabetes medications. His endocrinologist, initially skeptical, had been forced to acknowledge that something remarkable had happened - though she attributed it to "lifestyle changes" without understanding how profoundly different our approach was from the standard dietary advice she had given him for years.

Gerald's story illustrates how insulin dysfunction ripples through every hormone system - and how addressing the terrain can restore function that medications alone never could. But insulin is just one piece of the hormone puzzle. In the next chapter, we will explore another critical hormone axis that profoundly affects how we feel, function, and age: the adrenal hormones and the response to stress.

Key Takeaways

- Insulin sits at the top of the hormone hierarchy - when insulin function is impaired, every other hormone system suffers.
- Insulin resistance is not malfunction but a protective response - cells resist glucose because their mitochondria cannot process what they already have.
- Conventional diabetes treatment often worsens the underlying problem by forcing glucose into already-overwhelmed cells, driving disease progression.
- GLP-1 medications like Ozempic reduce the glucose load but don't fix the terrain, create dependency, and may cause problematic muscle loss.
- Addressing root causes - mitochondrial dysfunction, inflammation, omega fatty acid imbalance, gut health, and nutrient deficiencies - can restore insulin sensitivity and reverse Type 2 diabetes.

Chapter 7

The Estrogen Question

The Adrenal Hormones: When Stress Becomes the Problem

Patricia was 51 years old and exhausted in a way that sleep couldn't fix. She would drag herself out of bed each morning feeling like she hadn't rested at all, push through her day on caffeine and willpower, then crash on the couch by seven in the evening - only to lie awake at night with her mind racing, unable to fall asleep despite her bone-deep fatigue.

"I feel like I'm running on empty," she told me at our first meeting. "But it's not just tired. It's like my body has forgotten how to make energy. I used to be able to handle anything - work stress, family demands, late nights when I needed them. Now the smallest things overwhelm me. If my schedule changes unexpectedly, I fall apart. If I skip a meal, I get shaky and irritable. I can't handle any stress at all anymore."

Patricia was a paralegal who had worked in high-pressure law firms for twenty-five years. She had always prided herself on being the calm one in a crisis, the person everyone could count on when deadlines loomed and tempers flared. But over the past three years, something had changed. The resilience that had defined her was gone, replaced by a fragility she didn't recognize.

"My doctor tested my thyroid and said it was fine," she continued. "She tested my iron - fine. She offered me antidepressants, but I'm not depressed. I'm exhausted. There's a difference. I know something is wrong with me. I just can't get anyone to figure out what it is."

What Patricia was describing - the profound fatigue, the inability to handle stress, the wired-but-tired feeling at night - pointed clearly to a problem that conventional medicine often overlooks: dysfunction of the adrenal hormones, particularly cortisol. Her stress response system, after decades of chronic activation, had become dysregulated, and until we addressed that, no amount of sleep, coffee, or willpower was going to restore her energy.

The Stress Response System: Designed for Survival

Your adrenal glands sit on top of your kidneys, and despite being small - about the size of a walnut - they produce hormones that affect virtually every system in your body. The most important of these is cortisol, often called the "stress hormone." But this label, while accurate, undersells cortisol's importance. Cortisol is not just about stress. It is essential for life.[73]

Cortisol regulates your blood sugar, keeping it stable between meals. It controls inflammation throughout your body. It affects your immune function, your blood pressure, your sleep-wake cycle, and your ability to form memories. Without adequate cortisol, you cannot survive - which is why complete adrenal failure is a medical emergency.[74]

In a healthy person, cortisol follows a predictable daily rhythm. It peaks in the early morning, giving you the energy to wake up and start your day. It gradually declines through the afternoon and evening, reaching its lowest point around midnight when you should be deeply asleep. This rhythm - high in the morning, low at night - is essential for normal energy, mood, and sleep.

The stress response system also includes adrenaline (also called epinephrine) and noradrenaline, which provide the immediate "fight or flight" response to acute threats. When you encounter danger, these hormones surge instantly, increasing your heart rate, sharpening your focus, and preparing your muscles for action. This response evolved to help us survive encounters with predators and other immediate threats.[75]

The problem is that this system evolved for a world very different from the one we live in today. Our ancestors faced occasional acute stressors - a predator, a rival tribe, a natural disaster. Between these events, life was relatively calm. The stress response would activate, do its job, and then turn off, allowing the body to return to baseline and recover.

Cortisol and Your Nervous System: The Gas Pedal and the Brake

To understand how cortisol affects your entire body, it helps you to understand your autonomic nervous system - the part of your nervous system that runs automatically, without you having to think about it. This system has two branches that work like the gas pedal and brake in a car.[76]

The sympathetic nervous system is your gas pedal. When activated, it speeds everything up. Your heart beats faster. Your breathing quickens. Your muscles tense. Blood flow shifts away from digestion and toward your muscles. Your pupils dilate. You become alert, focused, ready for action. This is the "fight or flight" state - your body is preparing to face a threat or run from it.

The parasympathetic nervous system is your brake. When activated, it slows everything down. Your heart rate decreases. Your breathing deepens. Your muscles relax. Blood flows to your digestive system. You feel calm, relaxed, at ease. This is sometimes called "rest and digest" - the state where your body heals, repairs, and recovers.

In a healthy person, these two systems balance each other. You can rev up when you need to - to meet a deadline, handle an emergency, or exercise intensely - and then calm down afterward. The gas pedal and the brake work together, each active at the appropriate time.

Cortisol is intimately connected to this balance. When cortisol is chronically elevated, it keeps the sympathetic nervous system activated.[8] Your body stays in "gas pedal" mode even when there's no immediate threat. Your heart rate stays elevated. Your digestion stays suppressed. Your muscles stay tense. You remain in a state of constant alertness that was meant to last minutes, not months or years.

This is why people with adrenal dysfunction often have digestive problems - their parasympathetic system never gets a chance to activate properly, so digestion suffers. It's why they have trouble sleeping - their body can't shift into the calm state needed for restful sleep. It's why they feel anxious even when nothing threatening is happening - their nervous system is stuck in alarm mode.

Over time, this constant sympathetic activation exhausts the system. The body loses its ability to respond appropriately to either real threats or real safety. Some people become stuck in a state of constant low-level anxiety. Others swing between hyper-vigilance and complete exhaustion. The nervous system, like the adrenals themselves, becomes dysregulated - unable to find its natural balance.

Chronic Stress: The Modern Epidemic

Modern life has fundamentally changed the nature of stress. Instead of occasional acute threats followed by periods of recovery, we face constant, low-grade stressors that never fully resolve. Work deadlines, financial pressures, relationship conflicts, news cycles, social media, traffic - the list is endless. Our stress response system, designed for short bursts of activation, is now running continuously.

This chronic activation has profound consequences. When cortisol stays elevated day after day, it stops being helpful and starts causing harm. Chronically elevated cortisol raises blood sugar, promotes fat storage around the midsection, breaks down muscle tissue, suppresses immune function, impairs memory and cognitive function, and disrupts sleep.[20] Many of the health problems we associate with aging - weight gain, cognitive decline, weakened immunity, poor sleep - are actually consequences of chronic cortisol elevation.

But the story doesn't end there. The adrenal glands, like any system in the body, have limits. When they are asked to produce high levels of cortisol continuously, month after month and year after year, they eventually begin to falter. The daily rhythm becomes disrupted. Morning cortisol, which should be high, starts to decline. The system that was once hyperactive becomes sluggish and dysregulated.[19]

This progression - from high cortisol to dysregulated cortisol to low cortisol - is what many practitioners refer to as "adrenal fatigue," though this term is controversial in conventional medicine. The controversy is largely semantic. Whether we call it adrenal fatigue, HPA axis dysfunction, or cortisol dysregulation, the clinical picture is real and recognizable: people who once handled stress easily now fall apart at minor challenges, people who wake exhausted and can't sleep at night, people who have lost their resilience and vitality.

The HPA Axis: Where the Brain Meets the Adrenals

To understand adrenal dysfunction, we need to understand the system that controls it: the hypothalamic-pituitary-adrenal axis, or HPA axis. This is the communication pathway between your brain and your adrenal glands, and it determines how much cortisol your body produces.[77]

We discussed the hypothalamus and pituitary gland earlier when we explored the hormone hierarchy. As you may recall, these two structures in your brain act as the master control center for your entire endocrine system. The hypothalamus monitors conditions throughout your body and sends signals to the pituitary, which then directs individual hormone-producing glands - including the adrenals - to increase or decrease their output. This same command structure that controls thyroid and sex hormones also controls cortisol production.

When the hypothalamus perceives stress - whether physical, emotional, or psychological - it releases a hormone called CRH (corticotropin-releasing hormone). This signals the pituitary gland, which responds by releasing ACTH (adrenocorticotropic hormone). ACTH travels through the bloodstream to the adrenal glands, telling them to produce cortisol.

In a healthy system, cortisol then feeds back to the hypothalamus and pituitary, signaling them to reduce their output. This negative feedback loop keeps cortisol in the appropriate range - high enough to meet the body's needs, but not so high as to cause damage. It's an elegant self-regulating system.

But chronic stress can damage this feedback system. When cortisol is elevated for too long, the receptors that sense it become less sensitive - similar to the insulin resistance we discussed in the last chapter.[78] The hypothalamus and pituitary no longer respond appropriately to cortisol levels. The feedback loop breaks down. Cortisol production becomes erratic - sometimes too high, sometimes too low, often at the wrong times of day.

This HPA axis dysfunction is at the root of most adrenal problems. The adrenal glands themselves may be perfectly capable of producing cortisol. But the signaling system that tells them when and how much to produce has become dysregulated. This is why simply taking adrenal hormones often doesn't solve the problem - and can even make it worse by further suppressing the body's own regulatory mechanisms.

How Hormone Replacement Can Make Adrenal Problems Worse

This brings us to an important and often overlooked problem: hormone replacement therapy, when given to someone with underlying adrenal dysfunction, can actually make things worse. This is true not just for cortisol replacement, but for thyroid hormones, sex hormones, and other hormone therapies as well.[19]

The most direct example is cortisol replacement itself. When you take cortisol or cortisol-like medications (such as prednisone or hydrocortisone), your HPA axis senses the incoming hormone and reduces its own production. The hypothalamus releases less CRH, the pituitary releases less ACTH, and the adrenal glands become dormant. This is appropriate when the medication is short-term. But with prolonged use, the adrenals can actually shrink from disuse, making it increasingly difficult to stop the medication.

But even non-cortisol hormones can worsen adrenal function. Thyroid hormone replacement is a perfect example. Many people with adrenal dysfunction also have symptoms of low thyroid function - fatigue, weight gain, brain fog, feeling cold. If a doctor tests their thyroid and finds it borderline low, they may prescribe thyroid medication. But here's the problem: thyroid hormone increases metabolic rate, which increases the body's demand for cortisol.[79]

If the adrenals are already struggling, adding thyroid hormone can push them past their limits. The person may feel better briefly as their metabolism speeds up but then crash as their adrenals cannot keep up with the increased demand. They end up feeling worse than before - more fatigued, more anxious, less able to cope. The solution isn't more thyroid hormone; it's addressing the adrenal dysfunction first.

Sex hormone replacement can create similar problems. Estrogen, progesterone, and testosterone all interact with the HPA axis and cortisol metabolism.[19] When these hormones are given without addressing underlying adrenal dysfunction, they can create further imbalances. The body's hormone systems are interconnected - you cannot simply add one hormone and expect everything else to remain stable.

This is one of the main reasons hormone replacement therapy fails for so many people or works initially and then stops working. The underlying adrenal dysfunction was never addressed. The HPA axis remained dysregulated. And the added hormones, rather than restoring balance, created new imbalances that made the original problems worse.

The lesson here is critically important: adrenal function must be evaluated and addressed before starting any hormone replacement therapy. If the HPA axis is dysregulated, adding other hormones is like trying to tune a piano that's missing strings. You might make some notes sound better, but the overall result will still be discordant.

Adrenal Dysfunction and the Rest of Your Hormones

The adrenal glands don't operate in isolation. They are intimately connected with every other hormone system in your body, and when adrenal function becomes dysregulated, the effects ripple throughout your entire endocrine system.

Remember the hormone hierarchy and pregnenolone steal we discussed earlier in this book? Pregnenolone is the precursor to all steroid hormones - including cortisol, DHEA, testosterone, estrogen, and progesterone. When the body is under chronic stress and needs to produce large amounts of cortisol, it diverts pregnenolone away from other hormone pathways.[80] This is why chronic stress often leads to low testosterone in men and progesterone deficiency in women. The raw materials are being used for cortisol instead.

Thyroid function is also directly affected by cortisol. Elevated cortisol inhibits the conversion of T4 to active T3, leading to symptoms of low thyroid function even when thyroid hormone production is normal.[1] It also increases reverse T3, which blocks thyroid receptors. Many people with "thyroid problems" actually have cortisol problems that are impairing their thyroid function.

Insulin and cortisol have a complex relationship. Cortisol raises blood sugar, which triggers insulin release. Chronic cortisol elevation contributes to insulin resistance. And insulin resistance, as we discussed, affects virtually every other hormone in the body. The connections are circular and reinforcing - dysfunction in one system drives dysfunction in the others.

This interconnection explains why so many people with adrenal dysfunction have multiple hormone imbalances. They come in complaining of fatigue and discover they also have thyroid problems, or sex hormone imbalances, or blood sugar issues. These aren't separate conditions - they're all manifestations of the same underlying pattern of terrain dysfunction, with adrenal dysregulation often at the center.

Patricia's Real Problem

When I evaluated Patricia comprehensively, the picture that emerged was exactly what her symptoms suggested: severe HPA axis dysfunction after decades of chronic stress, compounded by terrain factors that made recovery difficult.

A four-point cortisol test - measuring cortisol at waking, noon, evening, and bedtime - revealed a severely flattened curve. Her morning cortisol, which should have been at its peak, was barely in the normal range. Her evening cortisol, which should have been low, was actually higher than her morning level. Her rhythm was essentially inverted - low when it should be high, elevated when it should be low. No wonder she couldn't wake up in the morning and couldn't sleep at night.

Her DHEA - another adrenal hormone that should be balanced with cortisol - was severely depleted. This suggested long-term adrenal strain. The adrenals had been prioritizing cortisol production for so long that DHEA had been sacrificed. Her pregnenolone was also low, confirming that the raw materials for hormone production were being funneled almost entirely into the stress response.

As expected, her other hormones showed the downstream effects. Her progesterone was nearly undetectable - classic pregnenolone steal. Her thyroid looked "normal" on standard tests, but her free T3 was at the bottom of the range and her reverse T3 was elevated - the pattern of cortisol-induced thyroid suppression. Her fasting insulin was elevated, suggesting the beginnings of insulin resistance driven by chronic cortisol elevation.

Her terrain was compromised in ways that made recovery harder. Her gut showed significant dysbiosis - not surprising, since cortisol suppresses digestive function and alters the microbiome.[81] Her inflammatory markers were elevated. Her omega fatty acid ratio was imbalanced at 14 to 1. Her vitamin D was low at 24 ng/mL, and her magnesium was depleted - both common in chronic stress, and both necessary for proper adrenal function.

The history was equally telling. Twenty-five years of high-stress work. A difficult divorce eight years ago. Caring for aging parents while working full-time. Never taking real vacations. Using coffee to power through fatigue rather than addressing it. Pushing through illness rather than resting. She had been withdrawing from her stress response system for decades without ever making deposits.

A Different Approach

Patricia's previous doctor had offered antidepressants, which wouldn't address her actual problem. Another practitioner had suggested adrenal glandulars and high-dose cortisol precursors - an approach that might provide temporary relief but could further suppress her body's own hormone production. Our approach was different: restore the terrain, support the HPA axis, and let the body's regulatory mechanisms heal.

The first priority was reducing the stress load. This meant both external stressors and internal ones. Patricia needed to make real changes to her work situation - not just "stress management" techniques, but actual reduction in demands. She negotiated reduced hours at work. She set boundaries with family members who had been relying on her to solve their problems. She learned to say no.

We also addressed internal stressors - the terrain factors that were keeping her body in a state of chronic alarm. She eliminated the Toxic Nine, which reduced the inflammatory burden on her system. We healed her gut, removing a major source of immune activation. We corrected her nutrient deficiencies, giving her body the raw materials it needed for hormone production and stress response.

Sleep became a non-negotiable priority. Cortisol rhythm is intimately connected to sleep-wake cycles, and you cannot restore normal cortisol patterns while sleep-deprived.[82] Patricia committed to a consistent sleep schedule - in bed by 10 PM, awake at 6 AM, no exceptions. We used targeted supplements to support sleep initially while her natural rhythms recovered.

We supported her adrenals with adaptogenic herbs - plants that help the body adapt to stress and restore HPA axis function. These included ashwagandha, which has been shown to reduce cortisol and improve stress resilience, and rhodiola, which supports energy without the stimulation of caffeine.[83] These are not quick fixes - they work gradually to restore normal function rather than overriding the body's regulatory mechanisms.

Critically, we weaned her off caffeine. This was difficult - caffeine had been masking her fatigue for years. But caffeine stimulates cortisol release, and continuing to use it would prevent her HPA axis from recovering.[84] The first two weeks without coffee were hard. But as her natural cortisol rhythm began to normalize, she found she had more real energy than caffeine had ever provided.

Patricia's Transformation

Adrenal recovery is not fast. The HPA axis takes time to reset, and the longer it has been dysregulated, the longer recovery takes. I told Patricia to expect three to six months before she felt significantly better, and up to a year for full recovery. She committed to the process.

The first changes were subtle. Within a few weeks, she noticed that she was falling asleep more easily at night. The racing thoughts that had kept her awake were quieting. She wasn't waking up at 3 AM as often. Sleep, which had felt impossible, was starting to feel natural again.

By two months, her morning energy was improving. She no longer felt like she needed to be scraped out of bed. The caffeine cravings had faded. She was waking up feeling - not energetic yet, but at least not destroyed. The trajectory was clearly positive.

After four months, she repeated her cortisol testing. The results showed significant improvement. Her morning cortisol had nearly doubled - still not optimal, but moving in the right direction. Her evening cortisol had dropped. The rhythm was beginning to normalize. Her DHEA was rising. The system was healing.

By six months, Patricia felt like a different person. "I have energy again," she told me. "Real energy - not caffeine energy, not pushing-through energy. I wake up and I actually want to get out of bed. I can handle things that would have flattened me six months ago. I feel like myself again - the self I thought I had lost forever."

Her other hormones had improved as well. Her progesterone had risen significantly as pregnenolone was no longer being diverted entirely to cortisol. Her thyroid markers had normalized - free T3 up, reverse T3 down - without any thyroid medication. Her insulin sensitivity had improved. By addressing the adrenals, we had allowed the entire endocrine system to rebalance.

"The biggest change," she reflected, "is that I have resilience again. I can handle stress. Not because I'm pushing through it or ignoring it, but because my body can actually respond to it and recover. That's what I had lost - the ability to bounce back. Now I have it again."

Patricia's story shows how chronic stress can dysregulate the entire hormone system - and how restoring adrenal function allows everything else to heal. But adrenal dysfunction is just one piece of the puzzle. In the next chapter, we will explore how sex hormones - estrogen, progesterone, and testosterone - become imbalanced, and why these imbalances are symptoms of deeper MILA dysfunction rather than problems to be solved with simple hormone replacement.

Key Takeaways

- Cortisol is essential for life, but chronic elevation causes widespread damage including weight gain, immune suppression, cognitive decline, and disrupted sleep.

- Your nervous system has two branches - the sympathetic (gas pedal) and parasympathetic (brake) - and chronic cortisol elevation keeps you stuck in gas pedal mode, preventing rest and recovery.

- The HPA axis, the communication system between brain and adrenals, becomes dysregulated with chronic stress, leading to cortisol patterns that are low in the morning and elevated at night.

- Hormone replacement therapy can worsen adrenal problems by increasing metabolic demands beyond what the adrenals can support - adrenal function should be addressed before HRT.

- Adrenal dysfunction affects all other hormones through pregnenolone steal, thyroid suppression, and insulin resistance.

- Recovery requires reducing both external stressors and internal terrain factors, supporting the body's own regulatory mechanisms rather than overriding them.

Chapter 8

Testosterone for Women

Sex Hormone Imbalance: A Symptom, Not a Cause

When estrogen, progesterone, or testosterone levels come back low on a lab test, most doctors focus on one question: how do we raise them? The assumption is that the low hormone level is the problem - fix the number, fix the patient. But this assumption misses the point entirely. Low sex hormones are not the disease. They are a sign that something deeper has gone wrong.

This chapter explores the specific mechanisms that cause sex hormone imbalances. We will examine how these hormones are made, what disrupts their production, and why they decline. Understanding these causes is essential because it shifts our focus from chasing hormone numbers to addressing the terrain dysfunction that created the imbalance in the first place. The hormones aren't the problem. Your Mitochondrial-Immune-Lymphatic Axis is dysfunctional to the point that your liver, your gut, and your fat tissue can't do their jobs, while your toxic burden continues to accumulate - that's the problem.

The Building Blocks: Cholesterol, Mitochondria, and Pregnenolone

All of your steroid hormones - cortisol, DHEA, testosterone, estrogen, and progesterone - are made from cholesterol.[13] This single fact has enormous implications that conventional medicine has largely ignored. Cholesterol is not the villain it has been made out to be. It is an essential molecule, so essential that your body manufactures it even if you consume none in your diet. Without adequate cholesterol, you cannot make adequate hormones.

This creates a troubling irony in modern medicine. Millions of people take statin medications to lower their cholesterol as much as possible. Statins are among the most prescribed drugs in the world, and doctors often aim for cholesterol levels that would have been considered dangerously low just decades ago.[79] Yet these same patients frequently develop symptoms of hormone deficiency - fatigue, low libido, muscle weakness, depression, cognitive problems - and are then prescribed hormone replacement or antidepressants. The possibility that their aggressively lowered cholesterol might be contributing to their hormone problems is rarely considered.

Research has shown that statin use is associated with lower testosterone levels in men and can affect sex hormone levels in women as well.[85] Low-fat diets, which were promoted for decades as heart-healthy, can have similar effects by reducing the raw material available for hormone production. The body needs cholesterol - not excessive amounts, but adequate amounts - to produce the hormones that regulate virtually every system.

The first step in hormone production is converting cholesterol to pregnenolone. This conversion happens inside the mitochondria - the same cellular powerhouses central to the MILA framework.[54] Cholesterol is transported into the mitochondria of cells in the adrenal glands and gonads, where enzymes on the inner mitochondrial membrane convert it to pregnenolone. This is why mitochondrial health is critical for hormone production. If your mitochondria are damaged or dysfunctional, the very first step of hormone synthesis is compromised.

Pregnenolone is called the "mother hormone" because all other steroid hormones derive from it. From pregnenolone, the body can make cortisol, DHEA, testosterone, estrogen, or progesterone - depending on what it needs most. People with chronic fatigue, fibromyalgia, and other conditions associated with mitochondrial dysfunction often have hormone imbalances precisely because the mitochondria that should be producing energy are the same mitochondria that should be initiating hormone production.

Pregnenolone Steal: When Stress Hijacks Your Sex Hormones

We introduced pregnenolone steal in the previous chapter on adrenal hormones, but its effects on sex hormones deserve closer examination. When your body is under chronic stress, cortisol production takes priority. The body diverts pregnenolone toward cortisol and away from sex hormones.[80] From an evolutionary standpoint, this makes sense - survival trumps reproduction. But in modern life, where stress is constant rather than occasional, this diversion becomes chronic.

This is the Cell Danger Response in action - when the body perceives an ongoing threat, the mitochondria shift their priorities from normal hormone production toward stress response. It's not just about cortisol stealing pregnenolone; the entire cellular machinery reprioritizes away from reproduction and toward survival.

The consequences are predictable. Progesterone drops first and most dramatically because it shares the most direct metabolic pathway with cortisol. Testosterone falls as DHEA - its precursor - becomes depleted. Estrogen may initially rise relative to progesterone (creating estrogen dominance), then eventually falls as the entire system becomes exhausted. The pattern depends on how long stress has been present and how depleted the system has become.

Progesterone: Why It Falls First

Progesterone is often the first hormone to decline under stress and understanding why reveals several important mechanisms. While progesterone is typically discussed as a women's hormone, men produce and need progesterone too - and its deficiency affects both sexes.

In women, progesterone production requires ovulation. In a normal menstrual cycle, the follicle that releases an egg transforms into the corpus luteum, which produces progesterone for the second half of the cycle.[86] If ovulation doesn't occur - a condition called anovulation - progesterone production is minimal regardless of what the ovaries are otherwise capable of. Anovulatory cycles become increasingly common in perimenopause, but they also occur in younger women under significant stress, with blood sugar dysregulation, or with thyroid dysfunction.

In men, progesterone is produced primarily in the adrenal glands and testes.[87] While men produce much smaller amounts than women, progesterone serves critical functions in male physiology. It acts as a precursor to testosterone - meaning low progesterone can contribute to low testosterone. It also helps balance the effects of estrogen in men, just as it does in women. And it has the same calming, GABA-enhancing effects on the male brain that it has on the female brain.

Progesterone is particularly vulnerable to pregnenolone steal because of its position in the steroid hormone pathway. The same precursors that make progesterone can be shunted toward cortisol production. Under chronic stress, the body consistently chooses cortisol - in both men and women. This is one reason chronically stressed men often have both low testosterone AND symptoms like anxiety and insomnia that reflect progesterone deficiency.

Progesterone also has a short half-life and must be continuously produced to maintain adequate levels. Unlike estrogen, which can be stored in fat tissue and released gradually, progesterone levels depend entirely on ongoing production. Any disruption to the production machinery immediately affects progesterone levels.

The consequences of progesterone deficiency extend beyond reproductive symptoms. Progesterone enhances GABA activity in the brain, producing calming effects.[88] Low progesterone contributes to anxiety, insomnia, and irritability in both sexes. In women, it leaves estrogen unopposed, contributing to heavy menstrual bleeding, fibroids, endometriosis, and breast tenderness. In men, low progesterone has been associated with prostate enlargement and may contribute to the anxiety and sleep disturbances that often accompany low testosterone.

Testosterone: What Drives It Down

Testosterone is essential for both men and women - contributing to libido, muscle mass, bone density, energy, and sense of well-being. Several specific mechanisms cause testosterone to decline.

Cortisol and testosterone have an inverse relationship. When cortisol rises, testosterone falls.[89] This happens through multiple mechanisms: cortisol directly suppresses the hypothalamic-pituitary-gonadal axis, reducing the signals that tell the testes and ovaries to produce testosterone. It also depletes DHEA, the precursor from which most testosterone is made. Chronic stress is one of the most common causes of low testosterone in both sexes.

Insulin resistance suppresses testosterone production in men while often increasing it in women - a pattern seen in polycystic ovary syndrome (PCOS). In men, elevated insulin reduces the production of sex hormone binding globulin (SHBG), which paradoxically can lower total testosterone while initially raising free testosterone. Over time, insulin resistance impairs testicular function directly, leading to lower production overall.[90]

Sleep deprivation dramatically reduces testosterone. Studies show that sleeping five hours per night instead of eight can reduce testosterone levels by 10 to 15 percent.[91] Testosterone production peaks during sleep, particularly during REM sleep. Chronic sleep restriction - common in modern life - chronically suppresses testosterone production.

Nutrient deficiencies impair testosterone synthesis. Zinc is essential for testosterone production; zinc deficiency directly reduces testosterone levels.[92] Vitamin D functions as a hormone itself and supports testosterone production. Magnesium affects testosterone bioavailability. These deficiencies are extremely common in the modern population.

The Aromatase Problem: When Testosterone Becomes Estrogen

One of the most important yet overlooked causes of hormone imbalance is excessive aromatase activity. Aromatase is an enzyme that converts testosterone into estrogen.[93] Some aromatase activity is normal and necessary - men need some estrogen, and women produce some estrogen through this pathway. But when aromatase activity becomes excessive, it creates a double problem: testosterone falls while estrogen rises.

Visceral fat tissue is a primary site of aromatase activity. The more visceral fat someone carries, the more aromatase they have, and the more testosterone gets converted to estrogen.[94] This creates a vicious cycle: low testosterone promotes fat gain, fat gain increases aromatase activity, increased aromatase further lowers testosterone. This is why overweight men often have low testosterone and relatively high estrogen, and why losing visceral fat often improves testosterone levels without any direct hormone intervention.

Inflammation increases aromatase activity. Inflammatory cytokines upregulate the aromatase enzyme, accelerating testosterone-to-estrogen conversion.[95] This is the immune component of MILA dysfunction directly affecting hormone balance. Chronic inflammation literally shifts the testosterone-estrogen ratio toward estrogen - one more reason why calming the immune system is essential for hormone restoration.

Insulin resistance also increases aromatase activity. Elevated insulin promotes fat accumulation and directly stimulates aromatase expression. The metabolic dysfunction that leads to diabetes is the same metabolic dysfunction that disrupts sex hormone balance.

Alcohol consumption increases aromatase activity, which is one reason heavy drinking is associated with low testosterone and gynecomastia (breast tissue development) in men. Even moderate alcohol intake can affect this pathway.

Estrogen Dominance: Not Just a Women's Problem

Estrogen dominance is typically discussed as a women's health issue, but it has become an increasingly serious problem for men as well. In women, estrogen dominance means estrogen is too high relative to progesterone. In men, it means estrogen is too high relative to testosterone. Both patterns cause significant health problems, and both are becoming more common.

In women, several mechanisms create estrogen dominance. Anovulation eliminates progesterone production while estrogen continues to be made. Chronic stress diverts pregnenolone toward cortisol, depleting progesterone more than estrogen. Fat tissue produces estrone - a weaker but still active estrogen - independent of ovarian function. The more fat tissue present, the more estrone is produced, contributing to estrogen burden even when ovarian estrogen production is declining.

In men, estrogen dominance typically results from excessive aromatase conversion of testosterone to estrogen, combined with impaired estrogen clearance. The result is a man with low testosterone, relatively high estrogen, and a collection of symptoms that are often dismissed or misattributed: gynecomastia (development of breast tissue), loss of muscle mass, increased abdominal fat, low libido, erectile dysfunction, fatigue, depression, and cognitive difficulties.[74]

Male estrogen dominance has reached epidemic proportions. Sperm counts in Western men have declined by more than 50 percent over the past 40 years.[96] Testosterone levels have been declining about 1 percent per year independent of age - meaning a 60-year-old man today has significantly lower testosterone than a 60-year-old man in 1980.[96] The causes are multifactorial: rising obesity rates increase aromatase activity, environmental xenoestrogens (synthetic or natural chemical compounds that mimic estrogen) add to estrogenic burden, sedentary lifestyles reduce testosterone production, and processed diets provide poor nutritional support for hormone balance.

Environmental estrogens - xenoestrogens - affect both sexes but may have particularly concerning effects on male development and fertility. These synthetic chemicals found in plastics, pesticides, and personal care products bind to estrogen receptors and exert estrogenic effects.[97] They don't show up on standard hormone tests, but they contribute to the total estrogenic load the body must manage. Boys exposed to higher levels of xenoestrogens in utero and during childhood may experience altered development, and adult men face ongoing exposure that compounds the problem.

The symptoms of estrogen dominance in women - heavy periods, breast tenderness, fibroids, weight gain around hips and thighs, mood swings, and PMS - often worsen in perimenopause even as estrogen levels are falling. This seems paradoxical until you understand that progesterone is falling faster. In men, symptoms may be attributed to "normal aging" or depression rather than recognized as hormone imbalance. In both cases, the solution isn't simply to manipulate hormone levels - it's to address the underlying causes: reduce visceral fat, decrease inflammation, support liver function, heal the gut, and reduce xenoestrogen exposure.

Estrogen Metabolism: How Your Body Clears Estrogen Matters

Estrogen simply doesn't disappear when the body is done with it. It must be metabolized and eliminated - and how this happens matters enormously for health. Think of it like recycling: estrogen can be broken down through different pathways, and some pathways produce safe byproducts while others produce harmful ones.[97]

The liver processes estrogen through three main pathways. The first pathway - the protective pathway - produces byproducts that are easily eliminated and may even have anti-cancer properties. The second pathway - the harmful pathway - produces byproducts that can damage DNA and are associated with increased cancer risk. The third pathway - the growth-promoting pathway - produces byproducts that are strongly estrogenic and stimulate cell growth.[80] The balance between these pathways - not just total estrogen levels - influences health outcomes.

What determines which pathway your body uses? Several factors. Cruciferous vegetables - broccoli, cauliflower, Brussels sprouts, cabbage - contain compounds that push estrogen toward the protective pathway.[45] This is one reason diets rich in these vegetables are associated with better hormone balance and lower cancer risk. Inflammation tends to push estrogen toward the harmful pathway. Obesity shifts metabolism toward the growth-promoting pathway. Nutrient status, particularly B vitamins and antioxidants, affects how efficiently the liver processes estrogen through any pathway.

Liver function is paramount. The liver performs the initial processing of estrogen, and a sluggish or overburdened liver cannot do this job efficiently. Alcohol consumption, medication burden, environmental toxin exposure, and fatty liver disease all impair estrogen processing. Someone with poor liver function may have relatively normal estrogen production but accumulate estrogen - and its harmful byproducts - because they cannot clear it effectively. The lymphatic system plays a critical role here too, as it must transport these metabolites away from tissues for processing and elimination.

The SHBG Factor: When Hormones Get Trapped

Sex hormone binding globulin (SHBG) is a protein produced by the liver that binds to sex hormones in the bloodstream. Hormones bound to SHBG are inactive - they can't enter cells or exert their effects.[98] Only free (unbound) hormones are biologically active. This means SHBG levels dramatically affect how much hormone is actually available to your tissues, regardless of what your total hormone levels show on a blood test.

High SHBG effectively reduces hormone availability. Someone can have normal total testosterone but low free testosterone because too much is bound to SHBG. Conditions that raise SHBG include hyperthyroidism, liver disease, estrogen therapy, and low caloric intake. Aging tends to increase SHBG, contributing to declining free hormone levels even when total levels appear adequate.

Low SHBG creates different problems. When SHBG is low, more hormone is free and active, which might sound beneficial but can lead to excessive hormonal effects and faster hormone clearance. Conditions that lower SHBG include insulin resistance, obesity, hypothyroidism, and high androgen states like PCOS.[98] Low SHBG is often a marker of metabolic dysfunction - the same insulin resistance that lowers SHBG also disrupts hormone balance through other mechanisms.

Understanding SHBG explains why two people with identical total hormone levels can have completely different symptoms. It also explains why addressing metabolic health - insulin sensitivity, liver function, thyroid function - often improves hormone symptoms without directly manipulating hormone levels.

The Estrobolome: Your Gut's Role in Estrogen Balance

Your gut microbiome directly affects estrogen levels through a collection of bacteria called estrobolome. These bacteria produce an enzyme called beta-glucuronidase that can reactivate estrogen that the liver has already processed for elimination.[99]

Here's how it works: the liver conjugates estrogen - attaching a molecule to it that makes it water-soluble and inactive - then excretes it into bile, which enters the intestines. If gut bacteria produce excessive beta-glucuronidase, they remove the conjugate, reactivating the estrogen. This reactivated estrogen gets reabsorbed into circulation instead of being eliminated in stool.[11]

Dysbiosis - an unhealthy gut microbiome - typically increases beta-glucuronidase activity, leading to estrogen recirculation and accumulation. This can contribute to estrogen dominance even when ovarian estrogen production is normal or low. Constipation worsens the problem by giving bacteria more time to reactivate estrogen before it can be eliminated.

This gut-estrogen connection is a perfect example of how the MILA axis affects hormones. The gut houses roughly 70 percent of your immune tissue, and dysbiosis triggers immune activation that contributes to systemic inflammation. The gut's lymphatic vessels - the lacteals - are responsible for transporting fats and fat-soluble hormones. When gut health fails, both immune function and lymphatic drainage suffer, creating conditions for hormone imbalance.

The Accumulating Toxic Burden

Beyond xenoestrogens, many other environmental chemicals disrupt hormone function. Some interfere with hormone production by damaging the mitochondria where steroidogenesis begins. Others block hormone receptors, preventing natural hormones from exerting their effects. Still others impair the liver enzymes responsible for hormone metabolism and clearance.[41]

Heavy metals like lead, mercury, and cadmium accumulate in tissues and interfere with hormone production and receptor function.[100] Pesticides and herbicides - even at levels considered "safe" - have documented endocrine-disrupting effects. These exposures are cumulative. Your current hormone status reflects not just current exposures, but a lifetime of accumulated burden stored in fat tissue and bone.

This toxic burden helps explain why hormone imbalances have become so much more common over the past several decades. Our grandparents were not exposed to the same chemical soup we navigate daily. Addressing this toxic load - through reducing ongoing exposure and supporting detoxification pathways - is essential for lasting hormone balance. We will explore this in detail in the Eliminate phase of the R.E.S.T.O.R.E. MILA protocol.

The mechanisms we've explored in this chapter - pregnenolone steal, anovulation, aromatase activity, impaired estrogen metabolism, SHBG imbalances, gut dysbiosis, and environmental toxins - all trace back to dysfunction in the Mitochondrial-Immune-Lymphatic Axis. Damaged mitochondria can't produce hormones properly. An overactive immune system drives inflammation that disrupts hormone balance. A congested lymphatic system can't clear hormone metabolites effectively. Sex hormone imbalances are consequences of this deeper dysfunction, not primary problems requiring direct hormone intervention.

This understanding has profound implications for treatment. In the next chapter, we'll examine what happens when conventional medicine ignores these causes and jumps straight to hormone replacement - and why that approach so often makes things worse before making them better.

Key Takeaways

- Sex hormone production begins in the mitochondria, where cholesterol is converted to pregnenolone - mitochondrial dysfunction directly impairs hormone synthesis.

- Progesterone falls first under stress because it shares a metabolic pathway with cortisol and requires ovulation, which stress disrupts.

- Testosterone is suppressed by cortisol, insulin resistance, sleep deprivation, and nutrient deficiencies - all modifiable factors.
- Excessive aromatase activity converts testosterone to estrogen, driven by visceral fat, inflammation, and insulin resistance.
- Estrogen dominance is usually a ratio problem - progesterone falling faster than estrogen - not simply excess estrogen.
- The liver metabolizes estrogen through pathways that produce protective or harmful metabolites depending on nutrient status, inflammation, and liver health.
- SHBG determines how much hormone is actually available to tissues - metabolic dysfunction alters SHBG and thus hormone availability.
- The gut microbiome's estrobolome can reactivate estrogen meant for elimination, contributing to estrogen accumulation when dysbiosis is present.

Chapter 9

The HRT Promise

The Hormone Replacement Trap

Veronica was 52 years old and had done everything right - or so she thought. When perimenopause hit her hard at 48, she had sought out the best care available. She found a physician who specialized in bioidentical hormone replacement therapy, had comprehensive testing done, and started on a customized regimen of estrogen, progesterone, and a small amount of testosterone. For the first eight months, it felt like a miracle.

"I felt like myself again," she told me. "The hot flashes stopped. I could sleep through the night. My brain fog lifted. My mood stabilized. I had energy. I told everyone who would listen that bioidentical hormones had saved my life."

But then things started to shift. Around the nine-month mark, Veronica noticed her breasts becoming tender again - a symptom she thought she had left behind. She started retaining water. Her mood, which had been so stable, became unpredictable. She gained eight pounds despite no changes to her diet or exercise. When she reported these symptoms to her hormone doctor, the response was to adjust her doses - a little less estrogen, a little more progesterone. It helped briefly, then the symptoms returned.

Over the next three years, Veronica's hormone regimen was adjusted dozens of times. More estrogen, less estrogen. Different forms of progesterone. Adding DHEA. Removing DHEA. Changing delivery methods from creams to pills to pellets. Each adjustment would provide temporary relief, then the symptoms would return - often worse than before. By the time she came to see me, she was on her fourth hormone doctor and feeling worse than she had before she ever started treatment.

"I don't understand," she said, frustrated and exhausted. "The hormones worked at first. Everyone said bioidentical hormones were safe and natural. Why did they stop working? What went wrong?"

What went wrong was that Veronica's hormone replacement had never addressed why her hormones were imbalanced in the first place. The treatment had masked her symptoms while the underlying dysfunction continued to worsen. She had fallen into what I call the hormone replacement trap - and she was far from alone.

The Promise and the Problem

Hormone replacement therapy - whether conventional or bioidentical - is built on a simple premise: if hormone levels are low, replace them. The logic seems unassailable. If a diabetic needs insulin, we give insulin. If a thyroid patient needs thyroid hormone, we give thyroid hormone. Why should sex hormones be any different?

The problem is that this logic ignores a fundamental question: why are hormone levels low in the first place? In Type 1 diabetes, the answer is clear - the pancreas has been destroyed by autoimmune attack and cannot produce insulin. The replacement is truly replacing something that cannot be made. But in most cases of sex hormone deficiency, the ovaries and testes are perfectly capable of producing hormones. Something else is suppressing their function or impairing hormone metabolism.

As we explored in the previous chapter, "something else" usually traces back to MILA dysfunction. Mitochondria can't efficiently convert cholesterol to pregnenolone. An immune system stuck in inflammatory overdrive that disrupts hormone signaling. A lymphatic system is too congested to clear hormone metabolites. A gut reactivates estrogen meant for elimination. A liver that's too burdened to metabolize hormones properly. When you add replacement hormones to this dysfunctional terrain, you're pouring water into a bucket full of holes.

The hormones may provide temporary relief because there are now more of them circulating. But the underlying dysfunction continues. The bucket keeps leaking. Eventually, the problems catch up - often manifesting as new symptoms that seem unrelated to hormone therapy but are actually direct consequences of it.

Why Hormone Replacement Works - At First

Understanding why hormone replacement often works initially - then stops working - requires understanding how the body responds to incoming hormones.

When you first start hormone replacement, you're adding hormones to a depleted system. The cells have been starved for these hormones and respond eagerly. Receptors that have been waiting for signals suddenly receive them. Symptoms that resulted from hormone deficiency - hot flashes, fatigue, brain fog, low libido - improve because the deficiency has been corrected. This honeymoon period can last weeks or months, and it feels like the treatment is working perfectly.

But several processes are happening simultaneously that eventually undermine the treatment. First, the body's own hormone production decreases through negative feedback. When the hypothalamus and pituitary sense adequate hormone levels - whether from your own production or from replacement - they reduce their signaling to the ovaries and testes.[101] Over time, this can lead to reduced natural production, making you increasingly dependent on replacement.

Second, the underlying dysfunction that caused the hormone imbalance continues to progress. If gut dysbiosis was causing estrogen recirculation, it's still doing that - now with more estrogen available to recirculate. If liver function was impaired, it's now struggling to metabolize both your body's hormones and the replacement hormones. If inflammation was driving aromatase activity, it's still converting testosterone to estrogen - including the testosterone you're taking as replacement.

Third, hormone receptors can become less sensitive over time when continuously stimulated - a phenomenon similar to insulin resistance.[102] The same dose that worked initially now produces less effect. The typical response is to increase the dose, which works temporarily but accelerates receptor desensitization. This is how people end up on escalating doses of hormones with diminishing returns.

The Testosterone Trap

Frank was 54 years old, a regional sales manager who prided himself on his work ethic and competitive drive. But over the past few years, that drive had been fading. He was tired all the time, struggling to focus in meetings, and had gained twenty pounds around his midsection despite his efforts at the gym. His libido, once dependable, had diminished significantly. His wife had noticed the changes and encouraged him to see a doctor.

"My primary care doctor tested my testosterone and said it was low," Frank told me. "He referred me to a men's health clinic. They did more testing and confirmed it - my total testosterone was 285, which they said was way below optimal for my age. They started me on testosterone injections, and they also gave me HCG to keep my testicles from shrinking. For a few months, I felt amazing."

The testosterone replacement therapy (TRT) had given Frank back his energy and drive. His workouts improved. His mood lifted. His libido returned. He became an evangelist for TRT, telling friends and colleagues that it had changed his life. But what Frank didn't mention - because he didn't initially connect it - was that he was also taking 40 mg of atorvastatin daily for his cholesterol, which his cardiologist had started him on three years earlier.

By his second year on testosterone, Frank's initial improvements had plateaued. His energy wasn't what it had been at the peak of his treatment. He had developed some breast tenderness - gynecomastia, his clinic called it - which they attributed to estrogen conversion and treated with an aromatase inhibitor. His blood pressure had crept up. His hematocrit had risen to the point where he needed regular blood donations to keep it in a safe range. And despite the testosterone, his belly fat wasn't budging.

"Now I'm on testosterone, HCG, an aromatase inhibitor, blood pressure medication, and I'm still taking the statin," Frank said. "I feel like I'm managing side effects of treatments for side effects. And honestly, I don't feel much better than I did before I started any of this. What's going on?"

What was going on was a cascade of interventions that had never addressed Frank's underlying problems - and in some cases, had made them worse.

The Statin Connection

Frank's case illustrates a connection that conventional medicine rarely acknowledges: the relationship between statin medications and hormone dysfunction. As we discussed in the previous chapter, cholesterol is the raw material from which all steroid hormones are made. When you aggressively lower cholesterol with statin medications, you reduce the substrate available for hormone production.[80]

Studies have shown that statin use is associated with lower testosterone levels in men.[96] This isn't surprising when you understand the biochemistry - less cholesterol means less raw material for testosterone synthesis. But this connection is rarely considered when a man on statins presents with symptoms of low testosterone. Instead, he's sent to a men's health clinic and started on testosterone replacement, treating the symptom while continuing the medication that's contributing to the cause.

Statins also impair mitochondrial function by depleting CoQ10, a critical component of the mitochondrial energy production chain.[13] Remember that the first step of hormone synthesis - converting cholesterol to pregnenolone - happens inside the mitochondria. When mitochondrial function is compromised, this conversion becomes less efficient even when cholesterol is available. Frank's statin wasn't just reducing his cholesterol; it was impairing the very cellular machinery responsible for hormone production.

The cruel irony is that many of the symptoms that lead men to seek testosterone replacement - fatigue, muscle weakness, cognitive problems, low motivation - are also side effects of statin medications.[79] A man experiencing these symptoms while on a statin might actually be suffering from statin side effects rather than true testosterone deficiency. But if his testosterone is tested and found to be low - which the statin itself may be causing - the solution offered is testosterone replacement rather than reconsidering the statin.

The Cascade of Interventions

Both Veronica and Frank experienced what I call the cascade of interventions - the pattern where each treatment creates new problems that require additional treatments, which create their own problems, and so on. This cascade is almost inevitable when hormone replacement is given without addressing underlying dysfunction.

For Veronica, the cascade looked like this: Estrogen replacement helped her hot flashes but overwhelmed her liver's ability to metabolize it, leading to estrogen accumulation. The accumulated estrogen caused breast tenderness and water retention. Her doctor reduced estrogen and added progesterone. The progesterone helped initially but was being converted to cortisol due to her unaddressed adrenal dysfunction, leaving her again with inadequate progesterone effects. More progesterone was added. Her gut dysbiosis - never addressed - continued to reactivate estrogen through beta-glucuronidase activity, keeping her in a state of relative estrogen excess no matter how her doses were adjusted.

For Frank, the cascade began before his testosterone treatment even started. His statin was impairing both his cholesterol availability and his mitochondrial function, contributing to his low testosterone. The testosterone replacement suppressed his body's own production while his underlying metabolic dysfunction - insulin resistance, inflammation, visceral fat - drove aromatase activity that converted his testosterone to estrogen. The aromatase inhibitor blocked this conversion but disrupted his hormone ratios in other ways. His rising hematocrit was a predictable response to testosterone therapy that required regular phlebotomy. Each intervention addressed a symptom while creating new problems.

This cascade is not a failure of the individual practitioners involved. Each intervention made sense in isolation. The problem is the paradigm itself - the assumption that hormone imbalances can be corrected by adding hormones, without addressing why the imbalances developed.

The Bioidentical Myth

Veronica had specifically sought out bioidentical hormone replacement, believing it would be safer and more effective than conventional HRT. This belief is widespread, but it reflects a misunderstanding of why hormone replacement often fails.

Bioidentical hormones are chemically identical to the hormones your body produces - as opposed to synthetic hormones like Premarin (derived from pregnant mare urine) or progestins (which are different from progesterone). This chemical identity does confer some advantages. Bioidentical hormones interact with receptors the same way your natural hormones do. They are metabolized through the same pathways. They don't have some of the problematic effects associated with synthetic hormones.[103]

But being bioidentical doesn't solve the fundamental problem. If your liver can't metabolize estrogen efficiently, it doesn't matter whether that estrogen is bioidentical or synthetic - it will still accumulate. If your gut bacteria are reactivating estrogen, they'll reactivate bioidentical estrogen just as readily. If your aromatase activity is elevated, it will convert bioidentical testosterone to estrogen just as it would any other form. The hormone may be identical to what your body makes, but if your body can't process it properly, problems will develop.

The bioidentical hormone movement has done valuable work in moving away from synthetic hormones and toward more physiological approaches. But it has not escaped the fundamental trap of treating symptoms rather than causes. A bioidentical hormone given to a person with unaddressed MILA dysfunction will eventually cause problems - perhaps different problems than synthetic hormones would cause, but problems, nonetheless.

Why the Body Reduces Its Own Production

One of the most significant consequences of hormone replacement is the suppression of the body's own hormone production. This happens through negative feedback - when the hypothalamus and pituitary sense adequate hormone levels in the blood, they reduce their signaling to the gonads.[101] This is why men on long-term testosterone replacement often experience testicular atrophy, and why stopping hormone replacement after extended use can be extremely difficult.

Frank's use of HCG was intended to prevent this. HCG mimics luteinizing hormone (LH), the signal from the pituitary that tells the testes to produce testosterone. By taking HCG alongside testosterone, the hope was to maintain testicular function and prevent atrophy. This approach is better than testosterone alone, but it doesn't fully solve the problem. The hypothalamus and pituitary are still receiving feedback that hormone levels are adequate, so they still reduce their natural signaling. The system becomes dependent on external inputs.

This dependency is one reason people often feel worse when they try to stop hormone replacement than they did before they started. Their own production has been suppressed, sometimes for years. The regulatory system has adapted to external hormones and doesn't immediately recover when those hormones are withdrawn. This creates a powerful incentive to continue replacing it indefinitely - you feel terrible without it, so you conclude you must need it.

But what often gets missed in this logic is that the person's own production was suppressed artificially. Their body didn't lose the ability to make hormones - it was told not to make them because external hormones were present. If the underlying dysfunction that caused the original hormone imbalance could be addressed, and the regulatory system given time to recover, many people could restore their natural hormone production. But this option is rarely explored because it requires a completely different approach than simply adjusting hormone doses.

When Replacement Creates New Imbalances

Hormone systems are interconnected in complex ways. When you add one hormone from outside, you inevitably affect the balance of other hormones - often in ways that aren't anticipated.

Estrogen replacement affects thyroid function by increasing thyroid-binding globulin (TBG), which binds more thyroid hormone and reduces the amount available to tissues.[1] Women who start estrogen replacement sometimes develop symptoms of low thyroid function even though their thyroid is producing adequate hormone. If this connection isn't recognized, they may be started on thyroid medication - another intervention to address a problem created by the first intervention.

Testosterone replacement affects estrogen levels through aromatase conversion - Frank's gynecomastia was a direct result of this. It can also affect red blood cell production (causing the elevated hematocrit that required Frank's blood donations), cholesterol levels, and liver function. Each of these effects can trigger additional interventions.

Progesterone replacement can affect cortisol pathways, GABA receptors, and other neurosteroid functions in ways that vary dramatically between individuals. What produces calm and improved sleep in one person can cause anxiety and insomnia in another, depending on their individual biochemistry and the state of their terrain.

These interconnections mean that hormone replacement is never as simple as replacing a single deficient hormone. You're always intervening in a complex, interconnected system. When the terrain is dysfunctional, these interventions often create ripple effects that lead to new problems requiring new interventions - the cascade we see over and over again.

Finding the Root Causes

When I evaluated Veronica and Frank comprehensively, looking beyond their hormone levels to assess their terrain, the patterns underlying their struggles became clear.

Veronica's gut testing revealed significant dysbiosis with elevated beta-glucuronidase activity - her gut bacteria were reactivating the estrogen her liver was trying to eliminate. Her liver function markers showed signs of congestion and impaired phase II detoxification. Her inflammatory markers were elevated. Her omega fatty acid ratio was highly imbalanced. And her cortisol pattern was dysregulated, with low morning cortisol suggesting adrenal involvement - likely contributing to her progesterone being shunted toward cortisol production rather than exerting its intended effects.

Frank's picture was equally revealing. His fasting insulin was elevated at 18 - he was insulin resistant, which was driving both his visceral fat accumulation and his elevated aromatase activity. His inflammatory markers were high. His liver enzymes were mildly elevated - likely from the statin, which can cause liver stress. His CoQ10 level was depleted - another statin effect that was impairing his mitochondrial function. And his cholesterol, which his doctors considered well-controlled at 158 total, was arguably too low for optimal hormone production.

Neither Veronica nor Frank had a simple hormone deficiency that could be corrected with replacement. They had complex terrain dysfunction that was manifesting as hormone imbalance. The hormones they were taking weren't fixing the problem - in some ways, they were masking it, allowing the underlying dysfunction to progress while creating new imbalances that required additional interventions.

A Different Approach

The path forward for both Veronica and Frank required a fundamental shift in thinking - from managing hormone levels to restoring the terrain that produces and processes hormones.

For Veronica, this meant gradually reducing her hormone doses while simultaneously addressing her underlying dysfunction. We worked on healing her gut, which reduced the bacterial reactivation of estrogen. We supported her liver's detoxification pathways with targeted nutrients. We addressed her inflammation through dietary changes and omega fatty acid rebalancing. We supported her adrenals so that her progesterone could do its job rather than being diverted to cortisol production.

The process wasn't quick or easy. There was a period of adjustment as her body recalibrated to lower hormone doses. But as her terrain improved, she needed less and less external hormone support. Her body began to process hormones more efficiently, so lower doses produced better effects. Eventually, she was able to discontinue her hormone replacement entirely - something she had been told would never be possible - and maintain her well-being through terrain support alone.

For Frank, the first priority was addressing his metabolic dysfunction - the insulin resistance that was driving his aromatase activity and fat accumulation. We also had a careful conversation about his statin. Given his depleted CoQ10, elevated liver enzymes, and the likelihood that the statin was contributing to his hormone dysfunction, he decided to discuss alternatives with his cardiologist. He ultimately transitioned to a more targeted approach to cardiovascular risk that didn't involve statins.

With his metabolic health improving and the statin burden removed, Frank's own testosterone production began to recover. We gradually reduced his testosterone dose while supporting his body's ability to produce its own. His need for the aromatase inhibitor decreased as his inflammation and visceral fat decreased. His hematocrit normalized. After eighteen months of terrain restoration, Frank was producing adequate testosterone on his own and had discontinued all hormone-related medications.

When Hormone Replacement Is Appropriate

This chapter focused on the problems with hormone replacement when underlying dysfunction is ignored. But I want to be clear: hormone replacement is sometimes necessary and appropriate. The goal is not to avoid hormones at all costs but to use them wisely, in the right situations, with full understanding of what they can and cannot do.

There are situations where the hormone-producing organs have been damaged or removed - surgical menopause after hysterectomy with oophorectomy, or testicular damage from injury, infection, or cancer treatment. In these cases, the body truly cannot produce adequate hormones, and replacement is necessary and appropriate. There are also situations where age-related decline has progressed to the point where restoration of natural production is unlikely, and careful hormone support can improve quality of life.

The key distinction is whether hormone replacement is the first intervention or the last resort. In the conventional approach, replacement comes first - and often comes without any investigation into why levels are low. In the terrain-based approach, replacement is considered only after underlying dysfunction has been addressed and natural production has been given the opportunity to recover.

We will explore these exceptions in more detail in the next chapter. But for most people with hormone imbalances - like Veronica and Frank - the path to lasting improvement runs through terrain restoration, not hormone replacement. The hormones were never the primary problem and replacing them was never going to be the solution.

Understanding when hormone replacement becomes a trap - and when it might be genuinely necessary - requires discernment and individualized assessment. In the next chapter, we'll explore the exceptions: the situations where hormone support is truly appropriate, how to distinguish them from cases where terrain restoration should come first, and how to use hormones wisely when they are needed.

Key Takeaways

- Hormone replacement often works initially because it provides hormones to a depleted system, but the underlying dysfunction that caused the depletion continues to progress.

- Over time, hormone replacement suppresses the body's own production through negative feedback, creating dependency on external hormones.

- Statin medications can contribute to hormone dysfunction by reducing cholesterol availability and impairing mitochondrial function - yet this connection is rarely considered when treating low testosterone.

- The cascade of interventions - where each treatment creates problems requiring additional treatments - is almost inevitable when hormone replacement is given without addressing MILA dysfunction.

- Bioidentical hormones are not immune to these problems; they are still external hormones being processed by a dysfunctional terrain.

- The path to lasting hormone balance usually runs through terrain restoration, not hormone replacement - addressing the gut, liver, inflammation, and metabolic dysfunction that underlie the imbalance.

- Hormone replacement is sometimes necessary and appropriate, but it should be a last resort after underlying dysfunction has been addressed, not a first-line treatment.

Chapter 10

The Cortisol Myth

The Exceptions: When Hormone Support Is Truly Necessary

The previous chapter may have left you with the impression that hormone replacement is always a trap to be avoided. That was not my intention. My purpose was to show why hormone replacement so often fails when underlying dysfunction is ignored - not to argue that hormones should never be used. The truth is more nuanced. There are situations where hormone support is not only appropriate but essential for health and quality of life.

This chapter explores those exceptions. We will examine the circumstances where the body truly cannot produce adequate hormones and replacement becomes necessary. We will discuss hormones like thyroid, insulin, and cortisol where replacement can be lifesaving. We will consider how to distinguish situations that call for terrain restoration from those that require hormone support. And we will address the question that many people facing age-related hormone decline ask: at what point does supporting hormones make more sense than trying to restore natural production?

The goal is discernment - not a blanket rejection of hormone therapy, but a clear understanding of when it helps and when it hinders.

When the Factory Is Gone

The clearest indication for hormone replacement is when the organs that produce hormones have been removed or destroyed. In these cases, the body literally cannot make the hormones it needs, and replacement is not optional - it is essential.

Surgical menopause is the most common example. When a woman undergoes a hysterectomy with bilateral oophorectomy - removal of the uterus and both ovaries - she loses her primary source of estrogen and progesterone production overnight. Unlike natural menopause, which occurs gradually over years and allows the body time to adapt, surgical menopause is abrupt and complete. The ovaries, which had been producing hormones just hours before surgery, are simply gone.[104]

Women who experience surgical menopause, before the age of natural menopause, face significant health consequences without hormone replacement. The sudden loss of estrogen accelerates bone loss, increasing osteoporosis risk dramatically. It increases cardiovascular risk. It can cause severe hot flashes, vaginal atrophy, and sexual dysfunction. It affects cognitive function, mood, and sleep. For these women, hormone replacement isn't about optimizing already-adequate levels - it's about providing hormones their bodies can no longer make at all.[105]

The same principle applies to men who have lost testicular function. Testicular damage from injury, infection such as mumps orchitis, torsion, or cancer treatment including surgery, radiation, or chemotherapy, can permanently impair testosterone production.[74] Unlike age-related testosterone decline, where the testes are still capable of production if properly supported, these men have sustained damage to the testosterone-producing Leydig cells themselves. No amount of terrain restoration will enable damaged or absent tissue to produce hormones.

For these individuals, hormone replacement is not a trap - it is a necessity. The question isn't whether to replace hormones but how to do so in a way that maintains physiological balance and minimizes side effects. Even here, terrain health matters. A woman on estrogen replacement will still benefit from good liver function to metabolize that estrogen properly. A man on testosterone replacement will still do better if his inflammation is controlled and his aromatase activity is not excessive. But the hormones themselves are essential and cannot be avoided.

Lifesaving Hormones: Thyroid, Insulin, and Cortisol

Some hormones are so essential to survival that their replacement, when truly needed, is not a matter of optimization but of staying alive. Thyroid hormone, insulin, and cortisol fall into this category. When production of these hormones fails completely, replacement is mandatory.

Thyroid hormone replacement is necessary when the thyroid gland has been removed surgically or destroyed by radioactive iodine treatment - common approaches for thyroid cancer or severe hyperthyroidism. It is also necessary in

Hashimoto's thyroiditis when autoimmune destruction has progressed to the point where the gland can no longer produce adequate hormone.[5] Without thyroid hormone, metabolism slows to dangerous levels. Severe hypothyroidism - myxedema - can be fatal. For these patients, levothyroxine or other thyroid hormone replacement is lifesaving, not optional.

However, it's important to distinguish complete thyroid failure from the much more common situation of suboptimal thyroid function. Many people have thyroid symptoms - fatigue, weight gain, cold intolerance, brain fog - with technically "normal" lab values. In these cases, the question of whether thyroid medication is appropriate is complex. Often, addressing underlying factors like inflammation, nutrient deficiencies, gut health, and adrenal function can restore normal thyroid function without medication. Thyroid medication given to someone whose thyroid is capable of functioning properly can suppress the gland's own production and create dependency. The key is accurate assessment of whether the thyroid itself is damaged or whether other factors are impairing its function.

Insulin replacement is absolutely essential in Type 1 diabetes, where the immune system has destroyed the insulin-producing beta cells of the pancreas. These individuals produce no insulin and will die without replacement - not in years but in days to weeks. There is no terrain restoration that can regenerate destroyed beta cells. Insulin is not optional; it is survival.

Type 2 diabetes presents a different picture. In most cases of Type 2, the pancreas is still capable of producing insulin -

often it produces more insulin than normal. The problem is insulin resistance, not insulin deficiency. For these individuals, the appropriate first approach is addressing resistance through diet, lifestyle, and terrain restoration. Adding more insulin to an already insulin-resistant system can worsen the underlying dysfunction. However, Type 2 diabetes can progress to the point where the beta cells become exhausted and damaged from years of overproduction, and insulin replacement may eventually become necessary even here.

Cortisol replacement is lifesaving in primary adrenal insufficiency, also known as Addison's disease. In this condition, the adrenal glands themselves are damaged - usually by autoimmune attack, infection, or hemorrhage - and cannot produce cortisol. Without cortisol replacement, these patients face adrenal crisis, a medical emergency that can rapidly become fatal. They must take hydrocortisone or another corticosteroid daily for the rest of their lives, with dose increases during illness or stress.

This is quite different from the HPA axis dysfunction we discussed earlier, where the adrenal glands are capable of producing cortisol but the signaling system has become dysregulated. In HPA axis dysfunction, the treatment is restoring normal signaling, not replacing cortisol. In fact, giving cortisol to someone with HPA dysfunction will further suppress their already-struggling regulatory system. The distinction between true adrenal insufficiency and HPA axis dysfunction is critical -

one requires lifelong replacement, the other requires restoration of natural function.

Understanding the Three Estrogens

Before discussing when estrogen replacement is appropriate, it helps to understand that "estrogen" is not a single hormone but a family of related hormones with different properties and effects. The three main estrogens in the human body are estradiol (E2), estrone (E1), and estriol (E3).

Estradiol is the most potent estrogen and the primary estrogen produced by the ovaries during reproductive years. It is responsible for most of the effects we associate with estrogen - breast development, regulation of the menstrual cycle, maintenance of bone density, cardiovascular protection, and effects on mood and cognition. When we talk about estrogen declining in menopause, we're primarily talking about estradiol. Most estrogen replacement therapy uses estradiol or compounds that convert to estradiol.

Estrone is a weaker estrogen that becomes the predominant estrogen after menopause. It is produced primarily in fat tissue through conversion of androstenedione by the aromatase enzyme - the same process we discussed in relation to male estrogen dominance. Estrone can convert to estradiol and vice versa. Because it is produced in fat tissue, obese individuals have higher estrone levels, which contributes to their increased risk of estrogen-related cancers.[95]

Estriol is the weakest of the three estrogens. It is produced in large quantities during pregnancy by the placenta and is present at much lower levels at other times. Because of its weak estrogenic activity, some practitioners prefer estriol for hormone replacement, believing it provides benefits with less risk. Estriol is often used in topical preparations for vaginal atrophy because it acts locally without significant systemic effects.

Understanding these distinctions matters for hormone replacement decisions. The type of estrogen used, the delivery method (oral, transdermal, vaginal), and the dose all affect outcomes. Oral estrogens pass through the liver and can affect clotting factors and inflammatory markers differently than transdermal estrogens. Different estrogen formulations may be more appropriate for different situations and different women.

Age-Related Decline: Protection or Problem?

One of the most nuanced questions in hormone medicine is how to think about the natural decline in hormones that occur with aging. Is this decline a problem to be corrected, or is it a protective adaptation that we should respect?

There are arguments on both sides. From one perspective, hormone decline with aging is pathological - a form of deficiency that causes the symptoms and diseases we associate with aging. Restoring youthful hormone levels, in this view, should restore youthful function and prevent age-related disease. This perspective drives much of the anti-aging hormone replacement industry.

From another perspective, hormone decline may be protective. Lower estrogen levels after menopause mean less stimulation of breast and uterine tissue, potentially reducing cancer risk. Lower testosterone and growth hormone may reduce cancer risk more broadly since these hormones promote cell proliferation. Some research suggests that individuals with lower hormone levels naturally may actually live longer, not shorter.[106]

The nuanced truth likely lies somewhere in between, and it connects directly to the MILA framework we've been discussing. Some degree of hormone decline with aging may be natural and even protective. But the rate and degree of decline we see in modern populations likely reflects accelerated MILA dysfunction - accumulated toxic burden, chronic inflammation, mitochondrial damage, and metabolic dysfunction - rather than healthy aging. A 50-year-old today typically has lower hormone levels than a 50-year-old did a century ago, and this probably isn't because our ancestors were less healthy.

This suggests that the appropriate goal is not forcing hormone levels to match those of a 25-year-old but rather supporting appropriate hormone function for healthy aging. For some, this can be achieved through terrain restoration alone. For others, particularly those with more advanced decline or more severe symptoms, careful hormone support may be warranted - not to create supra-physiologic levels, but to restore function that has declined beyond what terrain optimization can address.

When Restoration Is No Longer Realistic

One of the hardest clinical judgments is determining when natural hormone production can be restored and when that ship has sailed. There is no bright line, and the answer varies by individual, by hormone, and by the degree and duration of dysfunction.

Several factors suggest that restoration may be possible: younger age, shorter duration of hormone dysfunction, identifiable and correctable underlying causes, and hormone-producing organs that are still intact and functional. A 45-year-old woman with low progesterone due to stress and anovulation has an excellent chance of restoring normal production if the underlying factors are addressed. A 35-year-old man with low testosterone due to sleep deprivation, obesity, and chronic stress can often restore normal levels through lifestyle changes and terrain support.

Other factors suggest that replacement may be necessary: older age, longer duration of dysfunction, absence or severe damage to hormone-producing organs, and failure of adequate restoration attempts. A 60-year-old woman who is ten years past menopause is unlikely to restart ovarian estrogen production regardless of how healthy her terrain becomes. A man whose testosterone has been low for a decade despite excellent metabolic health and lifestyle may have Leydig cell dysfunction that won't recover.

The pragmatic approach is to optimize terrain first in almost all cases, observe the response, and then reassess. *Many people who appear to need hormone replacement turn out to need terrain restoration instead* - their hormone production improves once underlying dysfunction is addressed. Others have genuinely exhausted their capacity for natural production and benefit from careful hormone support. The key is not making that determination prematurely, before giving restoration a fair chance.

A Framework for Decision-Making

Given the complexity of these decisions, a systematic framework can be helpful. Here's how I approach the question of whether hormone support is appropriate for a given individual.

First, is the hormone-producing organ present and functional? If the ovaries have been removed, if the thyroid has been destroyed, if the pancreas can no longer make insulin - then hormone replacement is necessary. No amount of terrain optimization can make absent organs produce hormones.

Second, if the organ is present, what is causing the dysfunction? Is it inflammation? Nutrient deficiency? Toxic burden? HPA axis dysregulation? Insulin resistance? If identifiable causes exist, address them and give the body time to respond before concluding that replacement is needed.

Third, how severe are the symptoms and what is the risk of waiting? A woman with severe hot flashes that disrupt her sleep and quality of life may reasonably choose hormone support while simultaneously working on terrain, rather than suffering for months during restoration. Someone with mild symptoms and good quality of life can afford to take more time with a restoration-first approach.

Fourth, what is the individual's age and life stage? A 42-year-old with premature ovarian insufficiency has different considerations than a 58-year-old with typical menopausal transition. Younger individuals have more to gain from restoration and more years ahead to either benefit from or suffer consequences of their choices.

Fifth, what are the individual's values and preferences? Some people are deeply uncomfortable with taking external hormones and will work harder at terrain restoration. Others are suffering acutely and want relief now. Both perspectives are valid, and the right approach respects individual autonomy while providing accurate information about options and consequences.

If Hormones Are Needed: Using Them Wisely

When hormone support is determined to be appropriate, several principles help maximize benefits and minimize risks.

Use the lowest effective dose. Higher is not better with hormones. The goal is to relieve symptoms and protect health, not to achieve the highest possible levels. Start low, increase gradually if needed, and find the minimum dose that achieves the desired effect.

Choose delivery methods thoughtfully. Transdermal estrogen avoids the first-pass liver effect and is associated with lower clotting risk than oral estrogen.[78] Testosterone injections create peaks and troughs that some men tolerate poorly; creams or pellets may provide more stable levels. The route of administration matters as much as the hormone itself.

Continue supporting terrain even while on hormones. Hormone replacement works better when the body can process hormones properly. Good liver function, healthy gut, controlled inflammation, and adequate nutrients all improve outcomes whether someone is on hormones or not.

Monitor and adjust. Hormone needs change over time. Regular monitoring - both symptoms and laboratory values - allows for appropriate adjustments. Some people find they need less hormone support over time as their terrain improves. Others may need adjustments as they age or as their circumstances change.

Consider cycling or periodic reassessment. For some hormones in some situations, it may be appropriate to periodically reduce or discontinue replacement to assess whether natural production has recovered. This is not appropriate for everyone - someone without ovaries or with destroyed thyroid obviously cannot recover production - but for those whose organs are intact, periodic reassessment prevents unnecessary long-term dependency.

The Bigger Picture

Throughout this book, we have argued that hormone imbalances are usually symptoms of deeper dysfunction rather than primary problems. This remains true even in cases where hormone replacement is necessary. The woman who needs estrogen after surgical menopause still benefits from addressing her terrain - it will help her process the estrogen she takes and reduce her risk of complications. The man with genuine hypogonadism who needs testosterone replacement will have better outcomes if his metabolic health is optimized.

Hormone replacement, when truly needed, is not a failure. It is a recognition that the body sometimes cannot do everything on its own. We don't consider it a failure when someone with Type 1 diabetes takes insulin or when someone with Addison's disease takes cortisol. These are appropriate medical interventions for genuine deficiencies.

The failure is not in using hormones when they're needed. *The failure is in using hormones reflexively, without investigating why they're low, without addressing modifiable causes, and without considering whether restoration might be possible.* The failure is in treating hormone levels as the problem rather than as the signal that something deeper has gone wrong.

The R.E.S.T.O.R.E. MILA protocol that we will explore in the coming chapters addresses this deeper dysfunction. For most people, following this protocol will improve hormone function without requiring replacement. For those who ultimately do need hormone support, the protocol will improve their response to that support and reduce their risk of complications. Either way, addressing the terrain is the foundation of lasting hormone health.

We have now completed our exploration of why hormone imbalances occur and when various interventions are appropriate. In the next section of this book, we turn from understanding the problem to implementing the solution. The R.E.S.T.O.R.E. MILA protocol provides a systematic approach to restoring the terrain that underlies hormone health. We begin with the Reveal phase - the comprehensive assessment that uncovers the specific patterns of dysfunction driving your hormone imbalance.

Key Takeaways

- Hormone replacement is essential when hormone-producing organs have been removed or destroyed, such as surgical menopause, testicular damage, or destroyed thyroid tissue.

- Some hormones are lifesaving: insulin in Type 1 diabetes, cortisol in Addison's disease, and thyroid hormone after thyroidectomy cannot be replaced by terrain restoration.

- The three estrogens - estradiol, estrone, and estriol - have different potencies and effects; understanding these distinctions helps guide appropriate replacement choices.

- Age-related hormone decline may be partly protective and partly pathological; the goal is appropriate hormone function for healthy aging, not forcing youthful levels.

- The decision to use hormone support should follow a systematic framework: Is the organ present? What's causing dysfunction? How severe are symptoms? What are age considerations? What does the individual prefer?

- When hormones are needed, use the lowest effective dose, choose delivery methods thoughtfully, continue supporting terrain, and monitor regularly.

- Even when hormone replacement is necessary, terrain health matters - it improves hormone processing and reduces complications.

Chapter 11

R - Reveal

R - Reveal: Discovering the Root Causes

I need to tell you about Maureen. Not because her case was unusual, but precisely because it wasn't.

At 49, she had spent the last four years chasing her hormones. It started when perimenopause hit - the hot flashes, the irregular periods, the mood swings that seemed to come from nowhere. Her gynecologist ran a hormone panel and declared her estrogen was "low for her age." She started on bioidentical estrogen. It helped for about three months.

Then the symptoms returned, along with new ones. Her doctor added progesterone. Better for a few weeks, then worse again. A functional medicine practitioner tested her thyroid and found her TSH was "suboptimal" at 3.2. She started on thyroid medication. Her hair stopped falling out, but her energy never improved. Another practitioner tested her cortisol and found a "flattened curve." She began taking adaptogens and adrenal support. The anxiety decreased slightly, but the fatigue persisted.

"I've had my hormones tested seventeen times in four years," Maureen told me during our first consultation, pulling out a thick folder of lab results. "Estrogen, progesterone, testosterone, DHEA, cortisol, thyroid - all of them, multiple times. Every practitioner finds something 'off' and tries to fix it.

I'm now taking estrogen, progesterone, thyroid medication, DHEA, pregnenolone, and six different supplements for adrenal support. And I still feel terrible."

She was exhausted despite sleeping nine hours a night. Her joints ached constantly. She had gained twenty pounds that wouldn't budge despite careful eating and regular exercise. Her brain fog was so severe she had reduced her hours as a paralegal because she couldn't concentrate on complex documents anymore. And perhaps most frustrating, her original symptoms - the hot flashes and mood swings - were never fully resolved despite all the hormone interventions.

"Everyone keeps adjusting my hormone levels," she said, her voice heavy with frustration. "More estrogen, less estrogen, different forms of progesterone, higher thyroid dose, lower thyroid dose. But nobody has ever asked why my hormones are imbalanced in the first place. They just keep trying to force the numbers into range."

Maureen had stumbled onto the central truth that this entire book has been building toward: hormone imbalances are symptoms, not causes. Every practitioner she had seen was treating her hormone levels as the problem, adjusting doses and adding hormones in an endless game of biochemical whack-a-mole. But none had investigated why her body wasn't producing, metabolizing, or responding to hormones properly.

"Maureen," I said, "we're not going to start by testing your hormones again. We're going to start by understanding your terrain - the underlying dysfunction that's causing all these hormone imbalances. The R.E.S.T.O.R.E. MILA protocol begins with Reveal precisely because clarity must precede action. Guessing is expensive - both financially and physiologically. You've already proven that treating hormone levels without understanding root causes doesn't work."

What "Reveal" Actually Means

To reveal is to see clearly what's hidden. In the context of MILA dysfunction, this means identifying the unique combination of mitochondrial stress, immune imbalance, and lymphatic stagnation creating your symptoms. This isn't about collecting data for data's sake - it's about asking the right questions so you can implement the right solutions in the right sequence.

Most conventional medicine operates on a model I call "test-and-treat." Run labs. Find abnormalities. Prescribe medications that force markers back into "normal" ranges.[99] The problem? Normal ranges don't equal optimal function. You can have "normal" TSH with profound hypothyroid symptoms. "Normal" estrogen with severe menopausal complaints. "Normal" cortisol with crushing fatigue.[11]

The MILA framework shifts the question from "Are your numbers normal?" to "Is your system functioning?" These are fundamentally different inquiries. The first looks at static snapshots. The second examines dynamic processes - the flow of energy, the balance of immune responses, the clearance of cellular waste, and the terrain that either supports or undermines hormone production and metabolism.

The Art of Asking the Right Questions

Before ordering a single test, before recommending any intervention, the Reveal phase begins with the Dynamic Intake. Not the rushed ten-minute encounter typical of conventional medicine, but a deep exploration of your health history, symptom patterns, environmental exposures, and lifestyle factors.

The questions that matter most aren't the ones on standard medical intake forms. They're questions that illuminate function, not just diagnosis:

When did your symptoms begin, and what was happening in your life at that time? Symptoms rarely appear randomly. There's usually a trigger - a viral illness, a period of chronic stress, toxic exposure, a major life transition. Identifying that trigger reveals which MILA component failed first.

Were there toxin exposures - mold, chemicals, heavy metals, or infections - that preceded your decline?[6] Environmental factors are upstream drivers of MILA dysfunction. A patient who lived in a mold-infested home will have different terrain issues than one who worked with industrial chemicals or had chronic infections.

How do your symptoms fluctuate with stress, sleep, food, or menstrual cycles? Symptom patterns reveal which systems are under the most stress. Symptoms that worsen with stress suggest HPA axis dysfunction. Symptoms that improve with sleep point to glymphatic and lymphatic drainage issues. Food-triggered symptoms indicate gut-immune axis problems. Symptoms that fluctuate with menstrual cycles reveal hormone metabolism dysfunction.

Do you feel worse with detox attempts, exercise, or certain supplements? This is perhaps the most revealing question. Patients who crash after detox have drainage issues. Those who feel worse after exercise have mitochondrial dysfunction.[6] Those who react badly to methylation support have impaired detoxification capacity.

What is your energy like in the morning versus afternoon? Energy patterns throughout the day reflect cortisol rhythm, mitochondrial function, and blood sugar regulation.[6] Morning fatigue suggests cortisol insufficiency or poor sleep quality. Afternoon crashes indicate mitochondrial burnout or reactive hypoglycemia. Evening exhaustion with racing mind suggests sympathetic overdrive.

These questions don't just collect information - they reveal patterns. And patterns point toward root causes.

The Dynamic Intake: Your Personal Health Map

The R.E.S.T.O.R.E. MILA Protocol uses what I call the Dynamic Intake - an intelligent, adaptive questionnaire that captures what standard medical histories consistently miss. Unlike conventional intake forms that focus on diagnoses and medications, the Dynamic Intake is designed to be intuitive, asking the next questions based on your answers from the previous ones, allowing it to explore the terrain factors that create and perpetuate illness:

Toxic exposure history: Occupational chemicals, mold exposure, heavy metal sources, pesticides, plastics, personal care products, water quality, air pollution.[100] Most patients don't connect their symptoms to the toxic burden they've accumulated over decades - but the body remembers every exposure.

Infectious history: Not just acute infections, but chronic, persistent, or recurrent infections. Epstein-Barr virus. Cytomegalovirus. Herpes simplex. Lyme disease and co-infections. Parasites. Fungal overgrowth.[81] These infections don't just "happen" - they reveal a terrain that can't maintain balance.

Immune patterns: Frequent infections, slow wound healing, autoimmune diagnosis or family history, allergies, food sensitivities, inflammation markers.[34] These patterns illuminate whether the immune system is under-functioning, over-functioning, or confused.

Digestive function: Bowel movement frequency and quality, gas and bloating patterns, food reactions, acid reflux, nausea, appetite changes.[107] The gut is simultaneously your largest immune organ and a major lymphatic hub. When gut health fails, so does systemic immunity and detoxification - including hormone metabolism through the estrobolome.

Energy and cognitive function: Sleep quality, morning energy, afternoon crashes, exercise tolerance, brain fog, memory issues, concentration problems.[6] These reveal mitochondrial capacity and glymphatic clearance efficiency - both essential for hormone production.

Hormonal status: Menstrual cycle regularity, PMS symptoms, libido changes, temperature regulation, stress response patterns, sleep-wake rhythm.[108] Hormones don't create MILA dysfunction - they mirror it. But their patterns reveal which aspects of MILA need attention.

Emotional and stress history: Major life events, trauma, chronic stress periods, mood patterns, anxiety or depression, sense of safety.[109] The nervous system doesn't distinguish between physical and emotional threats. Chronic emotional stress creates the same terrain dysfunction as chronic toxin exposure - and directly impacts hormone production through the HPA axis.

The Dynamic Intake is called "dynamic" because it evolves as patients progress through the protocol. It's not a one-time snapshot but a living document that adapts and refines the clinical picture. What you notice changes as your awareness increases. Symptoms you thought were normal reveal themselves as significant. Connections between seemingly unrelated issues become clear.

Functional Testing Through the MILA Lens

Once patterns are identified through the Dynamic Intake, targeted testing reveals the biochemical landscape beneath the symptoms. But not all tests are created equal. The most actionable tests are those that illuminate function, not just static markers.

I use what I call the Fundamental Four - a core testing strategy that provides the foundation for understanding MILA dysfunction in any patient:

Comprehensive Nutritional and Metabolic Assessment (CNMA)

This comprehensive nutritional assessment evaluates vitamins, minerals, amino acids, fatty acids, organic acids, oxidative stress markers, and toxin indicators.[110] It's not just about identifying deficiencies - it's about understanding how nutrients affect mitochondrial function, antioxidant capacity, neurotransmitter production, and detoxification pathways.

The organic acids panel within the CNMA is particularly revealing for hormone patients. It shows:

Mitochondrial function markers: Citric acid cycle intermediates reveal whether cells are generating energy efficiently or stuck in anaerobic metabolism.[29] Remember - the first step of hormone synthesis happens inside the mitochondria. If mitochondrial function is impaired, hormone production suffers regardless of how much raw material is available.

Neurotransmitter metabolites: Markers reflecting dopamine, norepinephrine, and serotonin metabolism.[111] These don't just indicate neurotransmitter levels - they show whether your body can produce and metabolize them properly, which directly relates to mood symptoms often attributed to "hormone imbalance."

Detoxification indicators: Markers showing whether phase II liver detoxification is functioning.[112] Low levels suggest impaired conjugation - your liver can't package hormones for elimination, leading to the estrogen dominance and hormone recirculation we discussed in earlier chapters.

Oxidative stress markers: These markers illuminate the cellular damage that accumulates when antioxidant systems can't keep up with oxidative burden.[113] Oxidative stress directly damages hormone-producing tissues and impairs the enzymes that synthesize and metabolize hormones.

Methylation Panel

Methylation is the process of adding methyl groups to molecules - a simple reaction that underlies thousands of critical functions. It's how your body produces neurotransmitters, processes hormones, repairs DNA, creates antioxidants, and detoxifies chemicals.[114] *When methylation fails, everything downstream suffers - including hormone metabolism.*

The methylation panel reveals genetic variants that affect methylation efficiency, functional markers showing whether methylation is actually happening regardless of genetics, cofactor status for the nutrients that make methylation possible, and detoxification metabolites revealing whether liver detoxification pathways are balanced.[112]

For hormone patients, methylation status is particularly important because estrogen is metabolized through methylation-dependent pathways. Impaired methylation can lead to accumulation of harmful estrogen metabolites rather than protective ones - the difference between the "protective pathway" and "harmful pathway" we discussed in Chapter 8.

Comprehensive Gastrointestinal Assessment

The gut is simultaneously the body's largest immune organ and a major lymphatic hub.[81] When gut health fails, so does systemic immunity, neurotransmitter production, nutrient absorption, and detoxification capacity. For hormone health specifically, the gut houses the estrobolome - the collection of bacteria that metabolize estrogen.

The Comprehensive Gastrointestinal Assessment reveals microbiome diversity and balance, inflammatory markers indicating intestinal inflammation, digestive function including enzyme production and fat absorption, intestinal permeability markers, and short-chain fatty acid levels.[115]

Beta-glucuronidase is a particularly important marker for hormone patients. This enzyme, produced by certain gut bacteria, can deconjugate estrogen that the liver has already packaged for elimination - forcing it to recirculate rather than being eliminated. High beta-glucuronidase activity is a major contributor to estrogen dominance that no amount of hormone adjustment can correct.[116]

Food Sensitivity Panel

Food sensitivities are different from food allergies. Allergies are immediate IgE reactions. Sensitivities are delayed IgG reactions that can take 72 hours to manifest, making them nearly impossible to identify without testing.[117]

Why does this matter for hormone patients? Because every time you eat a food your immune system reacts to, you trigger systemic inflammation.[8] Chronic inflammation drives cortisol production through the HPA axis. Elevated cortisol means pregnenolone steal - your body diverts hormone precursors away from sex hormones toward stress hormones. Chronic food sensitivities can perpetuate hormone imbalance regardless of what hormone treatments you receive.

Seeing Without Testing: The Power of Observation

Here's the reality: not everyone can afford comprehensive functional testing. A full Fundamental Four panel represents a significant investment. That's a barrier for many people seeking help.

But here's what's empowering: the Dynamic Intake form is accessible to everyone. While there is a small administrative fee to maintain the system, this fee is fully reimbursed with your first purchase at RestoreMILA.com. This intelligent assessment tool, combined with careful observation of your body's signals, provides profound insight into your MILA status without requiring expensive laboratory testing.

Your body constantly communicates its state through visible signs. Learn to read them:

Dark circles under eyes: Not just from poor sleep. Dark circles indicate lymphatic congestion, particularly in the lymph nodes that drain the face and sinuses.[118] The darker and more persistent, the more significant the drainage problem.

Puffiness or edema: Fluid retention signals lymphatic stagnation. If your rings feel tight by evening, if sock marks persist long after removal, if your face looks puffy in the morning - your lymph isn't flowing.

Skin issues: Acne, eczema, psoriasis, rashes - these aren't just skin problems. They're signs your primary elimination organs are overwhelmed, forcing your body to push toxins out through the skin.[21]

Energy crashes after eating: Post-meal fatigue reveals mitochondrial dysfunction and potential blood sugar dysregulation.[68] Food should energize you, not exhaust you.

Chemical sensitivity: Reacting to perfumes, cleaning products, or exhaust fumes indicate phase II detoxification problems.[41] Your liver can't conjugate and eliminate environmental chemicals efficiently - and it probably can't process hormones efficiently either.

Temperature dysregulation: Always cold? Can't tolerate heat? Poor temperature regulation reveals mitochondrial insufficiency and thyroid-adrenal dysfunction - not necessarily thyroid disease requiring medication, but terrain dysfunction affecting thyroid function.

Body odor changes: Impaired detoxification.[4] When internal elimination pathways are blocked, the body recruits every possible exit route - including sweat and breath.

Maureen's Revelation

When I evaluated Maureen comprehensively - looking beyond her hormone levels to assess her terrain - the patterns underlying her struggles became clear.

Her Dynamic Intake revealed several critical factors her previous practitioners had missed. Her symptoms had begun not with perimenopause but two years earlier, following a renovation project that had exposed her to significant mold and construction chemicals. She had been constipated for years, having a bowel movement every two to three days at best. She crashed after every "cleanse" or "detox" she attempted. She reacted badly to methylated B vitamins. She couldn't tolerate exercise without days of recovery.

Her Fundamental Four testing confirmed what history suggested:

Her CNMA showed severely elevated pyruvate and lactate - her mitochondria were trapped in Cell Danger Response, unable to complete aerobic metabolism. Her glutathione was depleted. Her omega-3 levels were critically low while inflammatory omega-6 markers were elevated. Every marker pointed to cells in crisis mode.

Her methylation panel explained her reaction to methylated supplements - she had compound genetic variants that required careful, gradual methylation support rather than aggressive supplementation.

Her gastrointestinal assessment was revelatory. She had severe dysbiosis with elevated beta-glucuronidase activity - her gut bacteria were reactivating the estrogen her liver was trying to eliminate. No wonder her estrogen levels never stabilized despite careful dosing adjustments. Her gut was recycling estrogen faster than her practitioners could adjust her hormones.

Her food sensitivity panel showed reactions to fourteen foods she was eating regularly, triggering constant low-grade inflammation that kept her HPA axis activated and her cortisol elevated.

"I finally understand," Maureen said, tears streaming down her face as I explained her results. "My hormones were never the primary problem. They were the symptom of everything else that was wrong - the toxic exposure, the mitochondrial shutdown, the gut dysfunction, the food sensitivities. Everyone was trying to fix my hormones while ignoring everything that was causing them to be imbalanced in the first place."

She was right. Her body had been communicating all along. She just needed someone who spoke the language.

From Data to Direction

The Reveal phase culminates in synthesis - taking all the information from the Dynamic Intake, testing, and observation, and creating a personalized map of dysfunction.

This map answers three critical questions:

Where is energy blocked? Mitochondrial dysfunction shows up as fatigue, exercise intolerance, brain fog, temperature dysregulation, and poor stress tolerance. For hormone patients, it also shows up as inadequate hormone production - remember, steroidogenesis begins in the mitochondria.

Where is inflammation unresolved? Immune hyperactivation appears as food sensitivities, autoimmune markers, chronic infections, allergies, and elevated inflammatory cytokines. For hormone patients, chronic inflammation drives aromatase activity, pregnenolone steal, and receptor resistance.

Where is waste trapped? Lymphatic congestion manifests as puffiness, dark circles, skin issues, chronic infections, slow healing, and reactions to detox attempts. For hormone patients, it manifests as inability to clear hormone metabolites, leading to estrogen dominance and toxic metabolite accumulation.

The answers to these questions determine your starting point. This is precision medicine - not treating hormone levels with standard protocols but understanding individual dysfunction patterns and addressing them systematically.

Understanding your terrain through the Reveal phase creates the foundation for restoration, but knowledge without action changes nothing. The map is useless unless you follow it. In the next chapter, we enter the E phase - Eliminate - where the real work begins. You'll discover why elimination must start with drainage, not detoxification, learning the critical distinction between mobilizing toxins and actually removing them from the body. For hormone patients like Maureen, opening drainage pathways is essential before hormone balance can be restored - her gut needed to eliminate estrogen properly, her liver needed to clear hormone metabolites, and her lymphatic system needed to transport it all for processing.

Key Takeaways

- Healing begins with revelation - understanding the specific patterns of mitochondrial dysfunction, immune imbalance, and lymphatic stagnation creating your hormone symptoms rather than endlessly adjusting hormone doses without addressing root causes.

- The Dynamic Intake and Fundamental Four tests reveal why hormones are imbalanced - illuminating nutrient deficiencies that impair hormone synthesis, methylation problems affecting hormone metabolism, gut dysbiosis driving estrogen recirculation, and food sensitivities perpetuating inflammation.

- Even without expensive testing, your body constantly communicates dysfunction through observable signs - dark circles signal lymphatic congestion, post-meal fatigue reveals mitochondrial failure, chemical sensitivity shows impaired detoxification that affects hormone clearance.

- The Reveal phase prevents dangerous mistakes - aggressive hormone treatment with blocked drainage causes symptom worsening, supplementation without proper assessment triggers adverse reactions, and treating hormone levels without understanding terrain perpetuates the cycle of adjustment and decline.

- Understanding empowers action - once you comprehend why your terrain has failed and why your hormones are imbalanced as a result, you gain agency to restore function systematically rather than remaining trapped in endless hormone adjustments that never address the underlying dysfunction.

Wondering where you are in the R.E.S.T.O.R.E. process? Scan the code below to complete Dr. Thoma's Dynamic Intake and discover which phase of healing your body needs most right now.

Chapter 12

E - Eliminate

E - Eliminate: Opening the Pathways of Flow

Rosemary was 47 years old and convinced her hormones were destroying her life. This marketing director had spent the past three years cycling through hormone treatments that never seemed to work for long. "I've tried everything," she told me at our first meeting, her frustration evident. "Bioidentical hormones, different forms of progesterone, thyroid medication, even testosterone cream. Each one helps for a few months, then stops working or makes things worse."

Her symptoms read like a textbook of hormonal chaos. Heavy, painful periods that had her missing work. Breast tenderness so severe she couldn't exercise. Bloating that made her look six months pregnant by evening. Weight that accumulated around her hips and thighs no matter what she ate. Mood swings that strained her marriage. Insomnia that left her exhausted but unable to sleep. Brain fog that made her fear for her job performance.

"My hormone doctor keeps adjusting my doses," Rosemary continued, pulling out a bag of creams, pills, and supplements. "More progesterone, less estrogen, add DIM, try a different thyroid medication. But nothing sticks. And lately, I've been getting worse even though my lab values look better. How is that possible?"

I looked at her comprehensive history. Rosemary had a high-stress job with long hours. She ate what she thought was a healthy diet - whole grains, low-fat dairy, lots of salads with commercial dressings. She used conventional personal care products and lived in a home with new construction that had never been properly aired out. She had been on antibiotics repeatedly in her thirties for recurrent sinus infections. She was constipated, having a bowel movement every two to three days at best.

"Rosemary," I said, "I don't think your problem is that you need different hormones or better doses. Your problem is that your body can't process the hormones you're already making - or taking. Your liver is overwhelmed with toxins and can't metabolize estrogen properly. Your gut bacteria are reactivating estrogen that should be eliminated. Your lymphatic system is congested and can't clear the metabolites. You're not suffering from a hormone production problem. You're suffering from a hormone elimination problem."

Her eyes widened. "Nobody has ever talked to me about elimination. They just keep trying to balance my levels."

"That's the problem," I replied. "You can't balance hormones when the drainage pathways are blocked. Before we can address your hormone levels, we need to open pathways that allow your body to process and eliminate hormones properly.

This is the Eliminate phase of the R.E.S.T.O.R.E. MILA protocol - and for someone with your pattern of estrogen dominance, it's absolutely essential."

The Intention of the Eliminate Phase

The Eliminate phase is the foundation of the entire R.E.S.T.O.R.E. MILA protocol. Its intention is twofold: stop the flow of toxins into your body and open your drainage pathways so toxins can exit.[119] Without this foundation, nothing else in the protocol works properly.

The wellness industry has created an entire economy around "detoxification" - a market worth billions annually that promises transformation in a bottle. Health food stores dedicate entire aisles to detox products: liver cleanses, colon cleanses, heavy metal chelators, parasite purges, and green powders guaranteed to "eliminate toxic buildup." The promise is seductive - simple solutions to complex problems, quick fixes for years of accumulation.

But here's the fundamental problem these products never address: you cannot detoxify effectively while continuing to pour new toxins into your body, and you cannot mobilize stored toxins if your drainage pathways are blocked. It makes no sense to bail water from a sinking boat without first plugging the hole. And it makes no sense to force toxins out of storage when they have nowhere to go.

Your body already knows how to detoxify - it has been doing it since before you were born. What it needs is not more products to force toxin release. What it needs is for you to stop adding to the burden while opening the pathways so the toxins it is already trying to eliminate can actually exit.

The Danger of Out-of-Sequence Detoxification

I learned the importance of proper sequencing dramatically early in my career while working in a clinical laboratory. One afternoon, blood samples came through from students in a health sciences course who had all started an aggressive detox program together. Every single sample showed catastrophic results: severely elevated liver enzymes indicating acute hepatic injury, kidney markers suggesting renal failure, and metabolic derangements consistent with systemic toxicity.

I ran the controls - they were perfect. I reran the samples - same results. These were not lab errors. These students' bodies were in crisis.

These young, relatively healthy students had overwhelmed their elimination pathways by mobilizing toxins before their drainage systems could handle the load. The program was aggressive: high-dose chelators, powerful binders, liver "flushers" - all taken simultaneously with no preparation and no drainage support. They were sick - fatigue, nausea, body aches, brain fog - but believed these were "healing crises" and kept pushing through. They had no idea they were poisoning themselves.

My recommendation was immediate: stop the detox program. Most recovered quickly once they stopped, but some had lingering effects for months. This experience crystallized a truth I have seen repeated countless times: *if you mobilize toxins faster than your lymphatic system can clear them, your liver can conjugate them, your kidneys can filter them, and your bowels can eliminate them, you create an internal toxic crisis.*

The three pillars must be addressed in order.

The Three Pillars of Elimination

This phase typically lasts eight to twelve weeks and operates through three pillars that must be addressed in sequence. This order is not arbitrary - it reflects biological requirements that cannot be circumvented no matter how eager you are to feel better.

Pillar One: Stop the Toxins

Before you can eliminate what is already in your body, you must stop adding more. This means eliminating the Toxic Nine foods - sugar, wheat, corn, soy, dairy, peanuts, seed oils, alcohol, and chemical additives - that systematically destroy MILA function.[11] It also means reducing environmental toxic exposures from personal care products, household cleaners, air quality, and water. Any continued exposure undermines your progress. You cannot detoxify faster than you are being poisoned.

Pillar Two: Get Lymph Flowing

Your lymphatic system is your body's primary drainage network, collecting waste from every cell and tissue. But unlike your circulatory system, it has no pump.[118] It relies entirely on your activity to move fluid. Deep breathing, walking, hydration, and manual techniques create the pumping action that moves lymph through vessels and clears the pathways for toxin exit. Without flow, toxins have nowhere to go.

Pillar Three: Remove Toxins

Only after you have stopped adding toxins and opened drainage pathways can you safely support toxin removal. Targeted supplements - drainage remedies, binders, glutathione, and immunoglobulins - capture and escort toxins out of your body through now-open pathways.[120] Attempting removal before the first two pillars are addressed creates the toxic recirculation that makes people sicker.

Pillar One: Eliminating the Toxic Nine

The Toxic Nine foods must be completely eliminated - not reduced, eliminated - for the duration of the protocol. This is not a recommendation; it is a requirement. Any continued exposure undermines your progress.

The Toxic Nine includes:

Sugar in all forms, including honey, maple syrup, and "natural" sweeteners. Sugar feeds pathogenic bacteria, disrupts blood sugar regulation, directly impairs mitochondrial function, and triggers inflammatory cascades throughout the body.

Wheat and gluten-containing grains damage the gut barrier by triggering zonulin release, causing intestinal permeability even in people without celiac disease. Gluten also triggers immune reactions and neurological inflammation.[55]

Corn and corn-derived ingredients including corn syrup, cornstarch, and corn oil - almost universally genetically modified and contaminated with glyphosate. GM corn contains Cry proteins that damage mitochondrial function.[121]

Soy in all forms acts as a potent endocrine disruptor that interferes with thyroid function, sex hormone balance, and contains compounds that inhibit nutrient absorption and burden the liver.

Dairy from any animal contains proteins that trigger immune reactions in many adults, particularly casein A1 found in conventional dairy, contributing to inflammation, congestion, and digestive dysfunction.

Peanuts are highly susceptible to aflatoxin contamination, a potent mycotoxin that damages the liver and immune system. They also contain lectins that can irritate the gut lining.

Seed oils including canola, soybean, corn, sunflower, safflower, and grapeseed are highly processed, oxidized, and inflammatory, disrupting cellular membrane function and promoting oxidative stress.[123]

Alcohol in any amount is directly toxic to mitochondria and the gut lining, depletes B vitamins and glutathione, disrupts sleep architecture, and requires significant liver resources to process.

Chemical additives including artificial sweeteners, colors, and preservatives are synthetic compounds that disrupt the gut microbiome, trigger immune reactions, and must be processed by the liver as toxins.

Beyond Food: Environmental Toxin Reduction

Food is just one source of toxic exposure. The average person encounters hundreds of chemicals daily through personal care products, household cleaners, air quality, and water. Reducing these exposures is essential during the Eliminate phase.[124]

Personal care products are absorbed directly through your skin. Conventional shampoos, conditioners, lotions, deodorants, makeup, and fragrances contain endocrine disruptors, preservatives, and chemicals that add to your body's toxic burden. Switching to cleaner alternatives dramatically reduces this daily exposure.

Household cleaners release volatile organic compounds that you breathe. Many contain ingredients that damage the gut microbiome when inhaled or absorbed. Simple alternatives - vinegar, baking soda, castile soap - clean effectively without the toxic load.

Water quality matters enormously. Municipal water often contains chlorine, fluoride, pharmaceutical residues, and other contaminants. A quality water filter for drinking and cooking water removes many of these exposures.

Air quality, both indoor and outdoor, affects your toxic load. Indoor air is often more polluted than outdoor air due to off-gassing from furniture, carpets, building materials, and cleaning products. Air purifiers with HEPA and activated carbon filters reduce this exposure significantly.

Pillar Two: Getting Lymph Flowing

The lymphatic system is your body's sewage system, collecting cellular waste and debris from every tissue. It is also intimately connected to immune function - the lymph nodes filter lymph and house immune cells that monitor for threats. When lymph stagnates, waste accumulates and immune function suffers.[34]

Unlike your cardiovascular system, which has the heart as a central pump, the lymphatic system has no dedicated pump. Lymph moves through a combination of muscle contractions, breathing movements, and the one-way valves within lymphatic vessels.[231] Without active movement, lymph stagnates.

Four primary methods get lymph flowing:

Hydration is fundamental. Lymph is primarily water, and dehydration makes it thick and sluggish. Drinking half your body weight in ounces of pure water daily keeps lymph thin and flowing.

Deep breathing is the most powerful lymphatic pump in the body. The diaphragm's movement during deep breaths creates pressure changes that actively push lymph through the thoracic duct - the main lymphatic highway.[125] Three to five minutes of intentional deep breathing several times daily dramatically improves lymph flow.

Movement activates the muscle contractions that squeeze lymphatic vessels. Walking, rebounding, swimming, yoga - any movement helps. You don't need intense exercise; you need consistent movement. Ten to twenty minutes of walking daily provides significant lymphatic benefit.

Manual techniques directly stimulate lymphatic flow. Dry brushing before showering, using gentle strokes toward the heart, activates superficial lymphatic vessels.[126] Professional lymphatic drainage massage can be helpful for those with significant congestion.

Pillar Three: Supporting Toxin Removal

Only after the first two pillars are addressed - toxin intake stopped and drainage pathways open - can you safely support active toxin removal. Attempting this step prematurely is where most detox programs fail.

Four supplements work together to support the elimination process:

Drainage supplement: Enhances lymphatic movement and supports the organs of elimination - liver, kidneys, and bowels. Many people notice reduced puffiness, clearer sinuses, and improved energy within the first few weeks. Continue throughout the Eliminate phase and longer if lymphatic symptoms persist.

Glutathione: Called the "master antioxidant" because it is essential for nearly every detoxification process in your body.[29] It protects your cells from oxidative damage during the elimination process, supports your liver in processing toxins, and helps regenerate other antioxidants like vitamins C and E. Most people with chronic health issues have depleted glutathione levels. Supplementation in liposomal or S-acetyl form ensures optimal absorption. Continue throughout the entire protocol.

Binder: Attaches to toxins in your digestive tract and carries them out through your stool.[127] Without a binder, toxins released during elimination can be reabsorbed in your gut through a process called enterohepatic recirculation - making you feel worse rather than better. A good binder captures a wide range of toxins including heavy metals, mycotoxins, and environmental chemicals. Take at least two hours away from food, other supplements, and medications. Ensure you have one to two daily bowel movements before adding binders.

Immunoglobulin support: Provides concentrated immunoglobulins that bind to toxins, bacteria, and inflammatory compounds in your digestive tract. By calming immune reactions in the gut, it reduces food sensitivities and supports gut barrier function. May be discontinued when gut reactivity and food sensitivities resolve.

Practical Implementation

The Eliminate phase typically lasts eight to twelve weeks and follows a specific sequence designed to address the three pillars safely and progressively.

Weeks 1-2: Stop the Assault and Establish Flow

Completely eliminate the Toxic Nine foods - no exceptions, no cheating. Begin reducing environmental toxic exposures. Start hydration protocol. Begin drainage supplement, glutathione, and immunoglobulins. Start gentle movement of ten minutes walking daily and deep breathing exercises two to three times daily. Add dry brushing before showers.

Weeks 3-4: Enhance Drainage

Increase movement to 15-20 minutes daily. Add castor oil packs three times weekly. Ensure one to two daily bowel movements before adding binder - this is critical. Introduce binder at bedtime, away from other supplements. Consider professional lymphatic massage if needed and tolerated.

Weeks 5-8: Optimize and Maintain

Continue all practices and supplements as directed in your MILA report. Monitor energy, mental clarity, and digestion for improvement. Add gentle sauna therapy of 15-20 minutes, two to three times weekly, if drainage remains open and tolerated.

Weeks 9-12: Assess and Prepare

Complete MILA Progress Assessment to measure improvement. Evaluate readiness for transition to the nutrition chapter and Strengthen phase. Continue all foundational practices - they remain essential throughout the protocol and beyond.

When to Advance

You are ready to advance when you have completed eight to twelve weeks in the Eliminate phase, your MILA Progress Assessment shows improvement in your scores, you are tolerating the supplements well without significant detox reactions, you have one to two daily bowel movements, and you have consistently implemented the lifestyle practices.

Positive signs of progress include increased energy, improved mental clarity, better sleep, reduced puffiness, clearer skin, normalized digestion, and enhanced exercise tolerance. Most people notice these improvements gradually over the eight-to-twelve-week period.

Stay longer if you experience worsening fatigue, increased brain fog, headaches, nausea, body aches, anxiety, insomnia, or skin breakouts when attempting to progress. These warning signs indicate your drainage pathways are not fully open. If these symptoms occur, slow down - reduce binders, focus more on the first two pillars, and give your body more time.

The goal is never to force elimination. The goal is to create conditions where elimination happens naturally, safely, and sustainably.

Rosemary's Transformation

The first two weeks were eye-opening for Rosemary. Eliminating the foods she had believed were healthy - the whole grains, the low-fat dairy, the commercial salad dressings loaded with seed oils - required rethinking everything she knew about nutrition. But by week three, something began to shift.

"The bloating," she said at her one-month follow-up, "it's finally going down. I can actually button my pants in the evening. And I'm having a bowel movement every day now - sometimes twice. I didn't realize how constipated I had been for years."

By week eight, her breast tenderness had resolved - completely. Her periods, while still heavy, were significantly less painful. The mood swings that had strained her marriage were smoothing out. She was sleeping through the night. And remarkably, her hormone levels - which we had not yet addressed with any treatment - were beginning to normalize on their own.

At twelve weeks, Rosemary's transformation was remarkable. Her estrogen-to-progesterone ratio, which had been severely imbalanced, had improved by 40 percent without any hormone treatment. Her liver enzymes, which had been mildly elevated, were now normal. The puffiness in her face and hands that she had attributed to aging was gone. She had lost twelve pounds without counting calories - the weight her body had been holding as it struggled to dilute and store toxins it couldn't eliminate.

"I spent three years trying different hormone combinations," Rosemary reflected. "Different doses, different delivery methods, different doctors. And the answer wasn't in the hormones at all. The answer was in opening my drainage pathways so my body could actually process hormones properly. I wasn't suffering from a hormone production problem - I was suffering from a hormone elimination problem. Once we fixed that, my body knew exactly what to do."

With drainage pathways now open and the body's elimination systems functioning, we turn to what may be the most powerful intervention of all: food. What you eat determines whether your drainage pathways stay open or become congested again, whether your immune system calms or remains hyperactive, whether your mitochondria generate abundant energy or struggle under toxic burden. In the next chapter, Eat to Restore: Nourishing the Terrain, we will explore why each of the Toxic Nine foods systematically damages MILA function, the whole foods that nourish and support healing, and the practical strategies that make this way of eating sustainable for life.

Key Takeaways

- The Eliminate phase operates through three pillars that must be addressed in sequence: first stop the toxins coming in through Toxic Nine food elimination and reduced environmental exposures, then get lymph flowing through hydration, breathing, movement, and manual techniques, and finally support toxin removal with targeted supplements.

- You cannot detoxify effectively while continuing to pour new toxins into your body - eliminating the Toxic Nine foods stops the ongoing assault so healing can begin, plugging the hole before you try to bail water from the sinking boat.

- The lymphatic system has no central pump and relies entirely on your activity to move fluid - hydration keeps lymph thin, deep breathing creates the most powerful pumping action, movement activates muscle contractions, and manual techniques stimulate vessel flow.

- Four supplements work together to support toxin removal once drainage is open: lymphatic drainage supplement to enhance flow, glutathione for cellular protection, binders to capture toxins in the gut, and immunoglobulins to calm gut immune reactions.

- The Eliminate phase typically lasts eight to twelve weeks; advance when MILA scores improve, you tolerate supplements well, have one to two daily bowel movements, and experience increased energy and mental clarity; remain longer if you experience worsening symptoms when attempting to progress.

- The body knows how to detoxify - it has been doing it since before you were born - but it can only do so effectively when you stop adding toxins, open drainage pathways, and then support removal in that specific order.

Chapter 13

Eat to Restore

Nourishing the Terrain

Claire's food journal looked like a prison sentence. At her sixth appointment with a functional medicine practitioner, she was handed yet another elimination list. No gluten. No dairy. No eggs. No nightshades. No nuts. No seeds. No legumes. No grains. No sugar. No fruit. No caffeine. No alcohol.

She was already down to about twenty foods, mostly chicken, fish, and vegetables, and still feeling terrible. Her Hashimoto's antibodies remained elevated. Her thyroid medication doses kept climbing. Her joint pain persisted. Her energy never climbed above 4/10. Every meal had become a source of anxiety rather than nourishment.

Her immune system was still confused. Her terrain was still broken. But now she also had orthorexia - a pathological obsession with eating only "pure" or "safe" foods that had destroyed her quality of life.

Claire's problem wasn't that she was eliminating foods. It was that she was eliminating the wrong foods based on generic protocols rather than her individual biochemistry. She had removed eggs, nightshades, nuts, seeds, and legumes - all nutrient-dense whole foods - without any testing to confirm she actually reacted to them. Meanwhile, she was still consuming seed oils in restaurant meals, corn-derived additives in "compliant" packaged foods, and chemical preservatives she didn't even know what to look for.

"I'm doing everything right," she told me, her voice cracking with frustration. "I've eliminated everything anyone has ever told me to eliminate. My thyroid is still attacking itself. My hormones are still a mess. What else can I possibly remove?"

"Claire," I said gently, "the question isn't what else to remove. The question is whether you're removing the right things - and whether you're nourishing your body with what it actually needs to heal your thyroid and balance your hormones."

The Two-Part Approach to Nutritional Healing

Effective terrain restoration requires understanding that not all food elimination is created equal. There are two distinct categories:

Universal Elimination: The Toxic Nine. Certain foods have been so fundamentally transformed by modern agriculture, genetic modification, and industrial processing that they damage the MILA system in virtually everyone. These aren't arbitrary restrictions based on the latest diet trend. They are foods that did not exist in their current form until the last 50 to 150 years and have coincided with an unprecedented epidemic of chronic disease - including the thyroid and hormone disorders that have become so common. The Toxic Nine must be eliminated by everyone pursuing terrain restoration.

Individualized Elimination: Food Sensitivity Testing. Beyond the Toxic Nine, each person has unique reactivities based on their genetics, gut health, immune status, and exposure history. One person may react strongly to eggs while another tolerates them perfectly. One may have issues with nightshades while another thrives on tomatoes and peppers. These individual sensitivities can only be identified through proper testing, not through generic elimination protocols that remove dozens of foods "just in case."

This distinction is critical. The autoimmune protocol diet has helped thousands reduce symptoms, and its emphasis on nutrient-dense whole foods while removing inflammatory triggers makes biological sense. But when practitioners apply it as a blanket protocol, removing eggs, nightshades, nuts, seeds, and legumes from everyone regardless of individual reactivity, they often create nutritional deficiencies, psychological distress, and paradoxically worse outcomes.

Claire's previous practitioners had her eliminate over thirty foods based on protocol, not her specific test results. When we finally ran comprehensive food sensitivity testing, we discovered she reacted to only four foods beyond the Toxic Nine - and none of them were the eggs, nightshades, or nuts she had been avoiding for years. She had been unnecessarily restricting nutrient-dense foods while still consuming hidden sources of corn, soy, and seed oils in "compliant" products.

Food as Medicine vs. Food as Restriction

Food as medicine means nourishing the body with nutrients that support healing - amino acids for tissue repair, minerals for enzymatic function, fats for hormone production, and phytonutrients for antioxidant protection. It means removing genuine inflammatory triggers - both the universally problematic Toxic Nine and your individual sensitivities identified through testing. It means working toward food freedom, not permanent imprisonment.[128]

Food as restriction means treating food as inherently dangerous, living in fear of reactions, eliminating more and more items indefinitely based on suspicion rather than evidence, and measuring success by how little you eat rather than how well you feel.

The goal of terrain restoration isn't to help you survive on twenty foods forever. The goal is to eliminate what's genuinely harmful, identify your individual sensitivities through testing, heal your gut barrier, rebalance your immune system, restore proper hormone metabolism, and ultimately restore tolerance so you can eat a varied, enjoyable diet of whole foods without triggering autoimmune or hormonal responses.[129]

The Toxic Nine: Foods That Destroy the MILA System

The average American gets approximately 70 percent of their calories from nine food categories that systematically attack the terrain. Each one damages MILA function through specific mechanisms - and each one directly impacts hormone production, metabolism, and signaling. Understanding why these foods are universally problematic empowers you to make informed choices rather than following rules out of fear.

Sugar

For approximately 2.5 million years, our ancestors consumed sugar exclusively from whole food sources, totaling less than 5 pounds per person annually.[34] Today, the average American consumes 150 to 170 pounds of added sugar annually - roughly 42 to 47 teaspoons per day.[130] This represents a 3,000 percent increase that our biochemistry simply cannot handle.

Sugar directly damages mitochondria through glycation, creating Advanced Glycation End Products that trigger inflammation. It feeds pathogenic bacteria and Candida in the gut, disrupting the microbiome and weakening gut barrier integrity.[131] For hormone health specifically, sugar drives insulin resistance, which increases aromatase activity and estrogen production. It depletes B vitamins and magnesium essential for hormone synthesis. And it creates the inflammatory environment that triggers pregnenolone steal, diverting hormone precursors away from sex hormones toward cortisol production.

Wheat and Gluten-Containing Grains

Today's wheat isn't your grandmother's wheat. Modern wheat has been extensively hybridized and selectively bred since the 1960s

Green Revolution, resulting in varieties with dramatically altered protein structures and increased gluten content.

Gluten triggers zonulin release, opening intestinal tight junctions and creating leaky gut.[55] This allows undigested proteins into the bloodstream, triggering immune activation and chronic inflammation. For thyroid patients like Claire, this is particularly significant - the molecular structure of gluten resembles thyroid tissue, and the immune system can become confused, attacking the thyroid when it encounters gluten proteins that have leaked through a damaged gut barrier. This molecular mimicry is a primary driver of Hashimoto's thyroiditis.

Corn and Corn-Derived Ingredients

Around 92 percent of U.S. corn is genetically modified to produce its own pesticide or resist herbicides.[132] These genetic modifications insert bacterial DNA into corn, causing every cell to produce Cry proteins that puncture insect gut linings.[133] Research shows these proteins damage human intestinal cells too.

Corn is also the source of high fructose corn syrup, which overwhelms liver mitochondria, creates fatty liver disease, and generates massive oxidative stress. For hormone health, HFCS drives insulin resistance and the cascade of hormonal dysfunction that follows - elevated estrogen, depleted progesterone, and impaired thyroid conversion.

Soy

Over 94 percent of U.S. soy is genetically modified with extremely high glyphosate residues.[134] Unfermented soy contains phytates that block mineral absorption, protease inhibitors that impair protein digestion, and phytoestrogens that disrupt endocrine function.[135]

Soy isoflavones interfere with thyroid hormone production, slowing metabolism and impairing mitochondrial function.[136] For anyone with thyroid concerns - and thyroid dysfunction underlies many hormone imbalances - soy consumption directly undermines recovery. Traditional Asian cultures consumed soy only in fermented forms like miso and tempeh, in small quantities as condiments - vastly different from the unfermented soy protein isolates that dominate the modern Western food supply.[137]

Dairy

Approximately 65 to 70 percent of the global population loses the ability to digest lactose after weaning - this is actually the evolutionarily normal state. Modern dairy from Holstein cows contains A1 beta-casein, which breaks down into BCM-7, an opioid peptide that triggers inflammation and immune activation.[138]

Dairy drives insulin and IGF-1 production, which affects hormone balance throughout the body.[139] Conventional dairy also contains residues from hormones and antibiotics given to cows.[140] For hormone patients, dairy's impact on insulin, its inflammatory proteins, and its potential hormone residues make it a significant contributor to endocrine disruption.

Peanuts

Peanuts aren't nuts - they are legumes that grow underground, making them susceptible to aflatoxin, a carcinogenic mold that damages liver mitochondria and suppresses immune function.[41] Peanuts contain potent lectins that damage the gut lining and trigger autoimmune responses. They have also been extensively hybridized to increase oil content, inadvertently increasing allergenic proteins.[141] The liver burden from aflatoxin exposure directly impairs the liver's ability to metabolize hormones properly.

Seed Oils

Soybean, corn, canola, sunflower, safflower, and cottonseed oils now comprise 20 percent of American calories, up from nearly zero in 1900.[142] These oils are extracted with hexane, bleached, and deodorized, creating trans fats and oxidized lipids. They are loaded with omega-6 linoleic acid, which incorporates into mitochondrial membranes, making them fragile and dysfunctional.

The omega-6 to omega-3 ratio in traditional diets is approximately 2:1 to 4:1. Modern Western diets often reach 15:1 to 20:1, driven by seed oil consumption. This imbalance creates chronic inflammation that underlies virtually all chronic diseases - including the inflammatory hormone conditions we have discussed throughout this book. Seed oils drive inflammation, insulin resistance, and obesity while poisoning mitochondria at the molecular level.

Alcohol

Alcohol is metabolized into acetaldehyde, a toxin that damages mitochondrial DNA and depletes glutathione. It increases intestinal permeability, impairs lymphatic pumping, and disrupts sleep architecture. Even moderate drinking suppresses immune function, disrupts hormone production, and accelerates aging.

For hormone health specifically, alcohol increases aromatase activity, converting testosterone to estrogen. It impairs liver detoxification of hormones. It disrupts the HPA axis and cortisol rhythm. And it depletes the B vitamins and minerals essential for hormone synthesis. The International Agency for Research on Cancer classifies alcohol as a Group 1 carcinogen - the same category as tobacco and asbestos.

Chemical Additives

The average American consumes 140 pounds of food additives annually, up from just 2 pounds in 1960. Preservatives like BHA, BHT, and TBHQ directly damage mitochondrial membranes. Artificial colors trigger immune responses. Emulsifiers like polysorbate 80 and carrageenan destroy the gut's protective mucus layer. Artificial sweeteners disrupt the gut microbiome and insulin signaling - and many are known endocrine disruptors that directly interfere with hormone function.

The MILA Cascade and Hormone Disruption

The Toxic Nine creates a self-perpetuating cycle of destruction: inflammatory foods damage mitochondria, leading to reduced ATP production. This impairs immune cell function and lymphatic vessel pumping. Increased inflammation results, and congested lymphatics fail to clear inflammatory debris. The cycle perpetuates and intensifies.[143]

For hormone patients, this cascade has specific consequences. Damaged mitochondria cannot perform the first step of steroid hormone synthesis. Inflammation drives aromatase and pregnenolone steal. Congested lymphatics cannot clear hormone metabolites. The liver, overwhelmed by the toxic burden, cannot properly conjugate and eliminate hormones. The gut, with its damaged barrier and dysbiotic microbiome, reactivates hormones that should be eliminated. Understanding this cascade explains why simply "eating healthy" while continuing to consume these foods rarely produces the hormonal results people hope for.

Why Animal Product Quality Matters

Conventional livestock practices introduce hormones, antibiotics, pesticides, and inflammatory fat profiles that accumulate in humans through the food chain.[144]

Synthetic hormones given to livestock increase IGF-1 levels in consumers.[145] Estrogen implants in cattle contribute to estrogen dominance in those who consume the meat.[146] Over 80 percent of antibiotics sold in the US are used in livestock production, and regular consumption exposes humans to constant low doses that disrupt the gut microbiome and impair immune function.[147]

Choosing pasture-raised, grass-fed, and organic animal products eliminates these concerns while providing superior nutrition:[148] Two to five times more omega-3 fatty acids, higher CLA levels with anti-cancer properties, more vitamins A, E, and K2, and omega-6 to omega-3 ratios of 2:1 to 3:1 compared to 10:1 to 20:1 in grain-fed meat. For hormone patients, the difference in fat quality alone can significantly impact inflammatory status and hormone metabolism.

The Practical Protocol: What to Eat

This protocol is built entirely from whole, single-ingredient foods that humans have consumed for millennia. Every item on this list would be recognizable to your great-grandparents and requires no ingredient label because it IS the ingredient.[150]

Protein Sources

Eggs from pasture-raised hens provide nature's perfect protein with all essential amino acids, choline for liver function, and healthy fats for hormone production. Fish, particularly wild-caught fatty fish like salmon, mackerel, and sardines, provide omega-3 fatty acids essential for reducing inflammation and supporting hormone balance. Chicken, turkey, and other poultry from organic, free-range sources. Grass-fed beef and lamb provide iron, zinc, B12, and conjugated linoleic acid. Wild game like venison and bison with naturally balanced omega fatty acid profiles. Tree nuts - almonds, walnuts, pecans, macadamias - providing protein, healthy fats, and minerals.

Complex Carbohydrates

Steel-cut or rolled oats provide sustained energy and soluble fiber. Brown rice as a whole grain staple. Quinoa as a complete protein source. Sweet potatoes provide complex carbohydrates with excellent micronutrient density. Beans and legumes - black beans, lentils, chickpeas - provide fiber and plant protein. White potatoes for those with higher caloric needs.

Vegetables

Virtually unlimited. All leafy greens, cruciferous vegetables like broccoli, cauliflower, and Brussels sprouts that support estrogen metabolism through beneficial pathways. Root vegetables, squashes, and hydrating vegetables like cucumber and celery. Bitter greens like arugula and dandelion that stimulate bile production for hormone clearance.

Fruits

All berries have lower sugar content and high antioxidant levels. Citrus fruits, stone fruits, apples, pears, melons, and tropical fruits. The fiber in whole fruit slows sugar absorption and provides satiety.

Healthy Fats

Extra virgin olive oil as the primary cooking and dressing fat. Avocado oil for higher-heat cooking. Coconut oil for its unique medium-chain triglycerides. Ghee, which is often tolerated even by dairy-sensitive individuals. Animal fats from quality sources.

The 16:8 Intermittent Fasting Window

An essential component of this protocol is timing your meals within an eight-hour eating window, allowing your body a sixteen-hour fasting period each day.[151] This approach provides profound metabolic and hormonal benefits beyond simple calorie restriction.

When you eat, insulin levels rise. Insulin is a storage hormone that tells your body to store energy rather than burn it.[152] During the sixteen-hour fasting window, insulin levels drop significantly, allowing your body to shift from glucose-burning to fat-burning.[68] For hormone patients, this insulin sensitivity improvement is crucial - insulin resistance drives aromatase activity, estrogen dominance, and the entire cascade of hormonal dysfunction.

Extended fasting also triggers autophagy - your body's cellular recycling program. During autophagy, cells break down and recycle damaged proteins and dysfunctional mitochondria.[153] This housekeeping process is essential for cellular health and has been linked to improved hormone receptor sensitivity and better hormone signaling.

Important consideration: Women may do better with a slightly shorter fast of 14 to 15 hours due to hormonal sensitivities. If fasting triggers significant symptoms, work with your practitioner to modify the approach.

The Gluten-Free Trap

One of the most concerning trends is patients who switch to gluten-free products believing they have made a healthy choice, only to become even more inflamed and hormonally disrupted than before.

Gluten-free junk food is still junk food. Gluten-free products are typically made with refined rice flour, tapioca starch, potato starch, and corn starch - all high-glycemic, nutrient-poor ingredients that spike blood sugar.[154] They contain added sugars, seed oils, gums, emulsifiers, and additives. Many contain corn and soy derivatives, meaning patients have simply traded one member of the Toxic Nine for others.

In clinical practice, some of the most hormonally disrupted patients are those who proudly declare they have been gluten-free for years. They have replaced wheat bread with gluten-free bread made from refined starches and sugar, wheat pasta with rice pasta stripped of fiber and nutrients. They have eliminated one problem while dramatically increasing their consumption of refined carbohydrates - driving the insulin resistance that perpetuates their hormone imbalance.

Don't find gluten-free replacements. Move beyond the bread-and-pasta paradigm entirely.[5]

Claire's Transformation

Claire's nutrition during the protocol was simpler than her previous restrictions. She eliminated the Toxic Nine but kept the whole foods she had been unnecessarily avoiding. Her food sensitivity testing showed she actually tolerated eggs, nightshades, and most nuts. She reacted to only four foods beyond the Toxic Nine: almonds, cinnamon, black pepper, and shrimp. Previous practitioners had removed over thirty foods based on protocol, not her specific reactivity.

Within six weeks, her digestion improved dramatically. By month three, following the daily structure and 16:8 fasting window, her Hashimoto's antibodies had decreased by 40 percent. Her thyroid medication dose was reduced for the first time in years. Her joint pain was minimal. Her energy climbed to 6/10.

"I'm eating more food than I was before," she told me at her six-month appointment. "I'm eating eggs. I'm eating nightshades. I'm eating walnuts and pecans. And I feel better than I did on twenty foods."

Her twelve-month labs showed antibodies in the low-normal range. Her thyroid function had stabilized. Energy was consistently 8/10. Joint pain was gone.

Claire worked with a therapist specializing in orthorexia alongside her physical healing. "I had to grieve the time I lost to food fear and restriction. The physical healing was important, but the psychological healing was just as essential."

Food Freedom as the Goal

The ultimate success of terrain restoration isn't measured by how restricted your diet becomes - it's measured by how much food freedom you reclaim while maintaining health.

The Toxic Nine must be permanently eliminated. These aren't foods you'll "earn back" after healing. They're fundamentally incompatible with human health regardless of how well your terrain is functioning. But beyond the Toxic Nine, the goal is maximum variety and enjoyment of whole foods.

Some people will have individual sensitivities that require additional permanent eliminations. That's biological reality, not failure. But these should be identified through testing, not assumed through fear. Most people discover they can enjoy a wide variety of whole foods - far more variety than they had on restrictive generic protocols.

Claire's relationship with food transformed from enemy to ally, from restriction to nourishment, from fear to freedom. That's what terrain restoration makes possible: not just managing hormone imbalance but actually living fully again.

With drainage pathways open from the Eliminate phase and nutritional foundations now in place, your body is finally ready to address the immune dysregulation that perpetuates chronic hormone imbalance. In the next chapter, we explore the Strengthen phase - where we turn our attention to rebalancing the immune system that has been in overdrive for far too long. The immune system, once calmed from the burden of constant toxic assault and inflammatory foods, becomes ready for the targeted regulation that restores balance between defense and tolerance - and allows hormone systems to finally normalize.

Key Takeaways

- The Toxic Nine - sugar, wheat, corn, soy, dairy, peanuts, seed oils, alcohol, and chemical additives - must be eliminated by everyone pursuing terrain restoration; these foods have been fundamentally transformed by modern agriculture and processing, creating compounds that systematically damage the MILA system and disrupt hormone function.

- Beyond the Toxic Nine, individual food sensitivities should be identified through testing rather than assumed through generic protocols; eliminating eggs, nightshades, nuts, or other whole foods without testing often creates nutritional deficiencies and psychological distress without addressing actual triggers.

- Animal product quality matters enormously for hormone health; choosing pasture-raised, grass-fed, organic sources eliminates hormone residues, antibiotic exposure, and inflammatory fat profiles while providing superior nutrition.

- The 16:8 intermittent fasting window improves insulin sensitivity, triggers cellular cleanup through autophagy, and supports hormone balance; women may need a slightly shorter fasting window due to hormonal sensitivities.

- Gluten-free processed foods often worsen hormone imbalance by replacing one Toxic Nine member with others while adding refined starches that drive insulin resistance; the goal is whole foods, not gluten-free substitutes.

- The goal is food freedom through terrain restoration - permanent elimination of the Toxic Nine, individualized elimination based on testing, and maximum variety of whole foods that nourish rather than damage hormone function.

For a more thorough understanding of the nutrition that supports every phase of the R.E.S.T.O.R.E. protocol, I direct you to my book Eat to Restore, a comprehensive dietary guide for terrain restoration.

Chapter 14

S - Strengthen

Restoring Immune Intelligence

Janelle was 41 years old and had been told her immune system was attacking her ovaries. This veterinary technician had always been healthy until two years ago, when her periods became irregular, her energy crashed, and hot flashes started waking her at night. Her gynecologist ran labs and delivered devastating news: premature ovarian failure. Her FSH was elevated, her estrogen was low, and her anti-mullerian hormone - a marker of ovarian reserve - was nearly undetectable.

"They found antibodies against my ovarian tissue," Janelle told me, her voice trembling. "Autoimmune oophoritis. My immune system is destroying my ovaries. They said there's nothing to do except hormone replacement for the rest of my life and to accept that I'll never have children."

At 41, Janelle had hoped to start a family. Now she was being told her reproductive system was being systematically dismantled by her own immune cells. She had started on estrogen and progesterone replacement, which helped with the hot flashes and sleep, but did nothing to address the underlying autoimmune attack. Her antibody levels remained high. Her ovarian function continued to decline.

"I keep asking why," she continued. "Why is my immune system attacking my ovaries? Nobody can tell me. They just say it happens sometimes. But it didn't just happen - something triggered this. I was fine two years ago. What changed?"

As I reviewed her history, the pattern emerged. Two and a half years ago, Janelle had developed a severe case of mononucleosis - Epstein-Barr virus infection that had kept her bedridden for three weeks. She never quite recovered her energy afterward. Six months later, her periods became irregular. A year after that, she received the autoimmune diagnosis.

"Janelle," I said, "your immune system isn't randomly attacking your ovaries. It's confused. That Epstein-Barr infection triggered an immune response that never properly resolved. Your immune system stayed activated, inflamed, unable to distinguish between the virus it was fighting and your own tissues. The hormone replacement you're taking is necessary right now, but it's not addressing the root cause. We need to retrain your immune system - teach it to stop the attack."

Her eyes widened. "You mean this might be reversible?"

"I can't promise your ovarian function will fully recover - some damage may be permanent. But I can tell you that calming the autoimmune attack gives your body the best possible chance to preserve what function remains and potentially restore some of what's been lost. Your immune system doesn't need to be suppressed with drugs. It needs to be re-educated. That's what the Strengthen phase is designed to do."

The Intention of the Strengthen Phase

The S Phase - Strengthen - focuses on restoring immune intelligence. Its intention is not to boost or stimulate your immune system, but to teach it how to regulate itself - responding vigorously to genuine threats while tolerating harmless substances and, critically, recognizing your own tissues as self rather than enemy.[155]

Modern medicine - both conventional and functional - makes the same fundamental mistake about immunity: they assume more is better. Boost immunity. Strengthen defenses. Support immune function. The language reveals the underlying assumption - that chronic illness results from weak immunity requiring enhancement. This is precisely backward.

In chronic illness, the immune system isn't weak - it's dysregulated. It's overactive in ways that cause harm, underactive in ways that allow opportunistic infections, and fundamentally unable to tell friend from foe. For hormone patients like Janelle, this immune confusion manifests as autoimmune attacks on hormone-producing tissues - the thyroid in Hashimoto's, the ovaries in autoimmune oophoritis, the adrenals in Addison's disease, the pancreatic beta cells in type 1 diabetes.

The problem isn't insufficient immune response - it's unintelligent immune response. The solution isn't immune stimulation. It's immune modulation - teaching the immune system to regulate itself.

This phase typically lasts eight weeks and builds on the foundation established in the Eliminate phase. With drainage pathways open and toxic burden reduced, your immune system now has the space and resources it needs to rebalance. Attempting immune modulation before drainage is established - while lymphatic channels remain blocked and toxins continue accumulating - creates temporary improvement at best.

The Core Principle: Modulation, Not Stimulation

The distinction between modulation and stimulation is critical and often misunderstood, even by practitioners.

Immune stimulation increases immune activity across the board - more antibodies, more inflammatory chemicals, more cell mobilization. This is appropriate for someone with genuine immune suppression: advanced HIV, post-chemotherapy, certain genetic immunodeficiency conditions. For these patients, the immune system truly is too weak and needs boosting.

Immune modulation teaches the immune system to respond appropriately - increasing activity against genuine threats while decreasing inappropriate reactions to harmless substances and self-tissues.[156] It's not about more or less immune function; it's about smarter immune function. The goal is to develop an immune system that responds vigorously to genuine threats while tolerating the foods you eat, the environment you live in, and your own hormone-producing organs.

Supplements marketed as "immune boosters" - echinacea, elderberry, astragalus, medicinal mushrooms, high-dose vitamin C - can actually worsen autoimmune conditions, food sensitivities, and chronic inflammatory states. They amplify an already-excessive immune response, adding fuel to a fire that needs to be contained rather than fed. For someone like Janelle, whose immune system was actively destroying her ovarian tissue, immune boosting would accelerate the damage.

The Immune-Hormone Connection

The relationship between immune function and hormone health runs deeper than most people realize. Immune dysregulation doesn't just occasionally affect hormone-producing tissues - it fundamentally shapes hormone production, metabolism, and signaling throughout the body.

Inflammation drives aromatase activity. Aromatase is the enzyme that converts testosterone to estrogen. Inflammatory cytokines - the chemical messengers of immune activation - directly increase aromatase expression in fat tissue.[36] This is why chronically inflamed individuals often develop estrogen dominance regardless of their baseline hormone levels. The immune system is literally changing their hormone balance.

Inflammation triggers pregnenolone steal. When the immune system is chronically activated, the body prioritizes cortisol production to manage the ongoing "threat." This diverts pregnenolone - the master hormone precursor - away from sex hormone production and toward cortisol synthesis.[80] The result is depleted testosterone, estrogen, and progesterone, all because the immune system won't calm down.

Inflammation impairs thyroid conversion. The conversion of T4 to active T3 is inhibited by inflammatory cytokines.[31] Patients can have adequate T4 levels but remain functionally hypothyroid because inflammation is blocking the conversion. No amount of thyroid medication fully corrects this until the inflammation is addressed.

Autoimmune attack destroys hormone-producing tissues. In Hashimoto's thyroiditis, the immune system attacks the thyroid gland. In autoimmune oophoritis, it attacks the ovaries. In type 1 diabetes, it attacks insulin-producing beta cells. In Addison's disease, it attacks the adrenal cortex.[157] These aren't separate diseases - they're the same immune dysregulation manifesting in different target organs. Addressing the underlying immune confusion is essential for preserving remaining function.

Understanding Inflammation's Complete Lifecycle

Understanding immune intelligence requires understanding inflammation's complete lifecycle. Most people think of inflammation as a single event: something harmful shows up, the immune system attacks it, things calm down. But inflammation is actually a two-phase process, and chronic illness occurs when the second phase fails.

Phase One: Starting the Fire. When cells sense danger - infection, tissue damage, toxin exposure - they release inflammatory signals. These chemical messengers trigger the classic inflammatory response: increased blood flow, fluid buildup, and pain signaling. This phase is essential - without it, infections would overwhelm us, injuries wouldn't heal, and damaged tissues couldn't be cleared and replaced. But inflammation was never meant to continue indefinitely.

Phase Two: Putting Out the Fire. This is where chronic illness patients get stuck. Ending inflammation isn't simply waiting for it to fade away - it's an active process requiring specific chemical signals and cellular behaviors. Scientists discovered molecules called Specialized Pro-Resolving Mediators, or SPMs - including resolvins, protectins, and maresins.[158] These molecules, made primarily from omega-3 fatty acids, actively signal the body to stop inflammation. They tell immune cells to stop producing inflammatory chemicals, switch from attack mode to repair mode, and clear away debris.

Without enough of these resolution signals, inflammation never fully ends. The immune system stays activated. Tissues remain inflamed. Energy continues draining into immune activity rather than normal cellular function. And for hormone patients, the inflammatory environment continues driving aromatase activity, pregnenolone steal, thyroid conversion problems, and autoimmune attacks on hormone-producing tissues.

S Phase Lifestyle Practices

The S Phase continues everything from the Eliminate phase - hydration, deep breathing, movement, dietary elimination of the Toxic Nine - while adding practices specifically designed for immune regulation. These lifestyle factors either support or undermine the regulatory mechanisms we're trying to rebuild. Supplements alone cannot restore immune intelligence.

Light Exposure: The Master Immune Regulator

Morning sunlight is one of the most powerful signals for regulating immune function. It sets your circadian rhythm, which controls the timing of immune cell activity throughout the day, and triggers vitamin D production in your skin. Vitamin D is not just a vitamin - it's a hormone that directly modulates immune function, reducing autoimmune activity while enhancing appropriate immune responses.

Get 10 to 20 minutes of morning sunlight within 30 minutes of waking - go outside without sunglasses so your eyes receive the light signal. This isn't optional - light exposure is a primary driver of immune timing and regulation. Evening light reduction supports melatonin production and proper immune timing. The contrast between bright morning light and dim evening light establishes the circadian patterns that govern immune cell behavior.

Movement as Immune Medicine

Exercise is one of the most powerful immune modulators known - but the type and intensity matter enormously during immune restoration.[159] Gentle movement - walking, yoga, swimming, tai chi - supports lymphatic flow and promotes anti-inflammatory signaling. During this phase, avoid high-intensity exercise, which can trigger inflammatory flares in already-dysregulated immune systems.

Think of "movement" rather than "exercise" - the goal is circulation and lymphatic flow, not performance or calorie burning. Continue building toward 30 minutes of gentle movement daily.

Sleep Optimization

The immune system does critical repair work during deep sleep phases.[160] Maintain consistent sleep and wake times even on weekends - the immune system thrives on predictable rhythms. Create a dark, cool sleep environment. Avoid screens for at least one hour before bed. Sleep optimization supports the immune rebalancing that occurs during rest - disrupted sleep perpetuates immune dysregulation regardless of what supplements you take.

Stress Management

Chronic stress directly suppresses immune regulation while amplifying inflammatory responses.[161] The stress hormone cortisol, when chronically elevated, shifts immune function toward inflammation and away from regulation. This is one mechanism by which emotional stress triggers autoimmune flares and worsens hormone imbalance.

Practice the MILA deep breathing technique twice daily: Lie down on a flat surface and place one hand on your chest and one hand on your stomach. Take a regular breath and while exhaling, push down on your stomach to fully get the air out. Then take a slow deep breath in, filling up your stomach with air and focusing on pushing your hand up. Continue the slow deep breath and focus on filling up your groin with air. Continue breathing in until you fill up your chest and neck with air as well. Open your mouth and exhale - the air should come out naturally without forcing. Complete 5 deep breaths, 2 to 3 times daily.

Social Connection

Loneliness and social isolation are profoundly inflammatory - studies show isolated individuals have significantly higher inflammatory markers than those with strong social connections.[162] Human touch, meaningful conversation, and community belonging all signal safety to the immune system, promoting regulatory function over defensive activation. This isn't optional - it's biological necessity for immune restoration.

S Phase Supplements

The S Phase supplements target inflammation and immune debris that have accumulated. These four interventions work synergistically to clear the battlefield, provide resolution signals, modulate immune pathways, and support regulatory cell function. Follow the dosing on product labels and your personalized MILA report directions.

Systemic Proteolytic Enzymes

Proteolytic enzymes - when taken between meals on an empty stomach - enter the bloodstream rather than being used for digestion.[163] Once in circulation, they break down inflammatory debris, immune complexes, excess fibrin, and other protein-based inflammatory material.

Think of systemic enzymes as cleanup crews that clear the battlefield so the immune system can accurately assess the current threat level rather than continuously responding to accumulated historical damage. When inflammatory debris is cleared, the immune system can finally stand down from its chronic activation. For autoimmune hormone conditions, this clearing allows the immune system to stop seeing hormone-producing tissues as ongoing threats.

Key enzymes include serrapeptase, nattokinase, bromelain, and papain. Take at least 30 minutes before meals or 2 hours after, allowing them to enter circulation rather than being consumed in digestive processes.

Omega-3 Fatty Acids

EPA and DHA from fish oil serve as precursors to those critical SPMs - the molecules that actively resolve inflammation. Without adequate omega-3 fatty acids, the body literally cannot produce the chemical signals needed to turn off inflammation. It's like trying to stop a war when you can't communicate the ceasefire order.

Most Americans consume omega-6 fatty acids in vastly excessive amounts relative to omega-3s. Historical ratios were likely 2:1 or 4:1. Modern Western diets often reach 15:1 or even 20:1. This imbalance biases the immune system toward inflammation and away from resolution. Therapeutic doses typically range from 2 to 4 grams of combined EPA and DHA daily. Quality matters enormously - rancid fish oil is pro-inflammatory, defeating the purpose.

Advanced Inflammatory Support

This is a full-spectrum botanical formula designed to help the body maintain a healthy inflammatory response. It contains a naturally balanced matrix of plant-derived polyphenols, protective oils, and bioactive proteins that work together to support antioxidant defenses, cellular resilience, and immune balance.[164]

Unlike pharmaceutical anti-inflammatories which suppress symptoms without addressing underlying dysregulation, these botanical compounds work with the immune system's natural regulatory mechanisms. The formula includes compounds that affect multiple inflammatory pathways simultaneously, stabilize mast cells to reduce histamine release, and support the shift from inflammatory to regulatory immune activity.

Continued Glutathione Support

Glutathione, introduced in the Eliminate phase for detoxification, continues playing essential roles in immune regulation.[165] Beyond its antioxidant and detoxification functions, glutathione directly affects immune cell behavior. T-regulatory cells - the immune cells responsible for preventing autoimmune reactions and calming excessive immune responses - require adequate glutathione for proper function.

When glutathione is depleted, regulatory T-cell function suffers, allowing unchecked inflammatory and autoimmune responses. For patients like Janelle with autoimmune attacks on hormone-producing tissues, supporting glutathione is essential for restoring the regulatory cells that should be preventing the attack. Continue supplementation in liposomal or S-acetyl form throughout this phase.

Practical Implementation: Your S Phase Protocol

The Strengthen phase typically lasts eight weeks, though individual variation exists based on the severity and duration of immune dysregulation.

Weeks 1-2: Initial Shifts

Continue all Eliminate phase practices and supplements. Add S Phase supplements as directed. Add morning sunlight exposure of 10 to 20 minutes within 30 minutes of waking. Subtle changes begin as systemic enzymes start breaking down accumulated inflammatory debris. Some experience temporary worsening - increased joint pain, fatigue, or brain fog - as debris is mobilized and cleared. This typically resolves within days.

Weeks 3-4: Resolution Accelerates

More noticeable improvements emerge. Food reactions often begin diminishing in severity. Joint pain and muscle aches decrease measurably. Energy becomes more stable throughout the day. Sleep quality improves as nighttime inflammation decreases. For hormone patients, this is often when hormonal symptoms begin stabilizing - fewer hot flashes, more regular cycles, improved mood.

Weeks 5-6: Immune Memory Rewrites

The immune system begins "remembering" how to regulate itself rather than defaulting to overreaction. Foods that previously triggered reactions may become tolerable in small amounts. Environmental sensitivities often decrease. Inflammatory markers on lab testing often show significant improvement. Autoimmune antibody levels may begin declining. Patients report feeling "more like themselves" - cognitive function sharpens, mood stabilizes, physical capacity increases.

Weeks 7-8: Consolidation and Transition

The immune system has established new patterns of response. Gains consolidate and stabilize. Energy is notably improved from baseline. The foundation is prepared for the next phase - Turbocharge. Complete MILA Progress Assessment to measure improvement and evaluate readiness for transition.

When to Move Forward

You are ready to advance when you have completed eight weeks in the S Phase, your MILA Progress Assessment shows improvement in your scores, inflammatory symptoms have meaningfully decreased, food sensitivities have reduced, you are tolerating the supplements well, and you have consistently implemented the lifestyle practices. Energy should be notably improved from your Eliminate phase baseline.

Stay longer if immune symptoms remain significantly active - persistent food reactions, ongoing joint pain, continued inflammatory flares, or if autoimmune markers remain highly elevated. Some patients with severe or long-standing immune dysregulation need additional weeks. Attempting to advance before immune regulation is established leads to problems in the Turbocharge phase when we stimulate mitochondrial energy production - you cannot safely increase cellular metabolism in an inflamed system.

Janelle's Transformation

Eight weeks into the Strengthen phase, Janelle returned looking like a different person. The exhaustion that had aged her prematurely was lifting. The joint pain she had developed alongside her ovarian symptoms had resolved. And most remarkably, her hot flashes had decreased significantly - even though we hadn't changed her hormone replacement doses.

"I finally understand what happened," she said. "That Epstein-Barr infection didn't just make me tired - it triggered an immune response that never turned off. My immune system was attacking everything, including my ovaries. The hormone replacement was just patching the downstream damage while the attack continued. Now that we're calming the immune system, the attack is slowing down."

Her latest labs confirmed the clinical improvement. Her inflammatory markers had dropped significantly. Her anti-ovarian antibodies, which had been highly elevated, had decreased by 35 percent. Her FSH, while still elevated, had actually improved slightly - suggesting her remaining ovarian tissue was responding now that it wasn't under constant immune attack.

"I don't know if I'll ever be able to have children," Janelle reflected, tears in her eyes. "But for the first time in two years, I have hope. My body isn't my enemy anymore. My immune system isn't randomly destroying me. It was confused, and now it's learning to recognize me as me again. Whatever happens with my fertility, I know I'm giving my body the best possible chance."

Six months later, Janelle's antibodies had dropped to near-normal levels. Her ovarian function, while not fully restored, had stabilized - and she was able to reduce her hormone replacement doses. She didn't achieve the pregnancy she had hoped for, but she did achieve something valuable: an immune system that had stopped attacking her body, and the knowledge that she had done everything possible to preserve her remaining hormonal function.

With drainage established in the Eliminate phase and immune regulation achieved in the Strengthen phase, the foundation is prepared for the next step in the protocol. Your lymphatic system is flowing. Your immune system has learned to regulate itself. Inflammation is finally resolving rather than perpetuating. Now we can address what many patients consider the core of their struggle: energy. The mitochondria - those cellular powerhouses that have been locked in survival mode, diverting resources to immune defense rather than energy production - can finally come back online. In the next chapter, we explore the Turbocharge phase, where we directly support mitochondrial function and restore the cellular energy that makes hormone production possible.

Key Takeaways

- The immune system in chronic illness and hormone imbalance isn't weak - it's dysregulated, overreacting to harmless substances and self-tissues while often failing to address genuine threats; immune "boosting" typically worsens autoimmune hormone conditions by amplifying already-excessive responses.

- Immune dysfunction directly drives hormone imbalance through multiple mechanisms: inflammation increases aromatase activity, triggers pregnenolone steal, impairs thyroid conversion, and in autoimmune conditions, directly destroys hormone-producing tissues.

- Inflammation is a two-phase process requiring active resolution signals; without adequate omega-3-derived SPMs, inflammation cannot properly resolve regardless of what triggers are removed, perpetuating the immune-hormone dysfunction cycle.

- Four supplements work synergistically: systemic enzymes clear inflammatory debris, omega-3 fatty acids provide resolution signals, advanced inflammatory support modulates immune pathways, and glutathione supports regulatory T-cell function essential for preventing autoimmune attacks.

- Lifestyle factors including morning light exposure, gentle movement, sleep optimization, stress management, and social connection are essential components of immune restoration - not optional additions to supplement protocols.

- The S Phase typically lasts eight weeks; advance when inflammatory symptoms have meaningfully decreased, food sensitivities have reduced, and energy has notably improved; remain longer if immune dysregulation persists to avoid problems when increasing cellular energy production in the Turbocharge phase.

Chapter 15

T - Turbocharge:

Restoring Mitochondrial Power

Lillian was 52 years old when she walked into my office, exhausted from carrying the weight of failed treatments. A former marathon runner and now a corporate trainer, she had been essentially housebound for the previous eight months. "I can barely make it from my bed to the kitchen," she said, her voice barely above a whisper. "I used to run 26 miles. Now I can't walk to the mailbox without needing to rest."

Her decline had begun three years earlier, coinciding with what she initially thought was perimenopause. The fatigue, brain fog, and mood changes seemed like normal menopausal symptoms. Her gynecologist agreed and started her on hormone replacement - estrogen and progesterone. She felt better for about six months.

Then the fatigue returned, worse than before. Her doctor added testosterone. Brief improvement, then decline. A functional medicine practitioner tested her thyroid and found suboptimal levels. She started thyroid medication. Another temporary boost, then crash. More hormones were added - DHEA, pregnenolone, adrenal support. Each intervention followed the same pattern: initial improvement lasting weeks to months, then a crash that left her worse than before.

"I've seen six practitioners in three years," Lillian explained, pulling out a shopping bag containing seventeen supplement bottles and four prescription medications. "They all focused on my hormones. They tested them, replaced them, balanced them, optimized them. And I kept getting worse. My last doctor said my hormone levels are now perfect - all in optimal ranges. But I can barely function. How can my hormones be perfect when I feel like I'm dying?"

I reviewed her extensive lab work. She was right - her hormone levels looked excellent on paper. Estrogen, progesterone, testosterone, thyroid, cortisol, DHEA - all carefully adjusted to fall within optimal ranges. Yet she was profoundly ill.

"Lillian," I said, "your hormones aren't the problem. They're the symptom. The real issue is that your mitochondria - the power plants inside every cell - have shut down. They're not producing the energy your cells need to function, including the energy needed to make and respond to hormones. You can replace hormones all day long, but if your cells can't produce the energy to use them, it doesn't matter what your levels are."

Her eyes widened. "So, all these hormones I've been taking..."

"They're like putting premium fuel in a car with a broken engine. The fuel quality is perfect, but the engine can't burn it. We need to fix the engine first. That's what the Turbocharge phase is designed to do - restore the mitochondrial function that makes everything else possible, including hormone production and hormone response."

The Intention of the Turbocharge Phase

The T Phase - Turbocharge - represents a critical inflection point in the R.E.S.T.O.R.E. MILA protocol. After opening drainage pathways in the Eliminate phase, establishing nutritional foundations, and achieving immune regulation in the Strengthen phase, the terrain has fundamentally shifted. Lymphatic flow has been restored. Toxic burden has decreased. Inflammatory cytokines have normalized. The immune system has remembered how to regulate itself. The stage is finally set for what patients desperately wanted from the beginning but couldn't safely receive: direct mitochondrial support.

This sequencing is not arbitrary - it reflects biological law. Mitochondria are exquisitely sensitive biosensors, constantly evaluating their environment for signals of safety or danger. When they detect threats - whether toxins accumulating in tissues, inflammatory cytokines flooding the extracellular space, or lymphatic stagnation preventing waste clearance - they initiate the Cell Danger Response, shifting from efficient energy production to defensive survival mode.

Attempting to force mitochondrial activation while danger signals persist doesn't boost energy - it triggers oxidative stress, inflammatory flares, and deeper fatigue. This is why Lillian and countless others crashed on hormone and supplement protocols. Their practitioners weren't wrong that energy was central to their illness. They were wrong about the approach - trying to force energy production without first creating the conditions where mitochondria feel safe enough to produce it.

The Core Principle: Cell Danger Response

Before exploring how to restore mitochondrial function, we must understand why it fails in the first place. The conventional view treats mitochondrial dysfunction as simple mechanical failure - cofactor deficiencies, oxidative damage, genetic mutations. While these factors matter, they miss the fundamental dynamic: mitochondria don't just break down randomly. They shut down intelligently in response to environmental threats, initiating a coordinated protective program called the Cell Danger Response.[29]

Think of the Cell Danger Response as your cellular emergency broadcast system. When mitochondria detect danger - whether from infections, toxins, nutrient deficiency, psychological stress, or chronic inflammation - they simply don't produce less ATP. They actively reorganize cellular priorities, shifting from growth and energy production to survival and defense. This involves multiple coordinated changes:

Metabolic shift: Energy production switches from oxidative phosphorylation - the efficient process generating 36 ATP per glucose - to glycolysis, which generates only 2 ATP per glucose.[166] This produces far less energy but allows cells to survive in hostile conditions. *Your energy crashes not because your* *mitochondria are damaged but because they have deliberately downshifted into survival mode.*

Hormone resistance: Cells reduce their responsiveness to hormones, particularly thyroid hormones and insulin.[18] This creates the pattern of "normal" hormone levels on lab tests while patients experience profound hormonal symptoms. The hormones are present, but cellular receptors are closed - another protective mechanism. This is why Lillian's perfect hormone levels translated to zero improvement. Her cells couldn't hear the hormonal signals because they were in defensive lockdown.

Steroidogenesis impairment: The first step of steroid hormone synthesis - the conversion of cholesterol to pregnenolone - happens inside the mitochondria.[13] When mitochondria are in Cell Danger Response, this conversion slows dramatically. You can have all the cholesterol raw material in the world, but if your mitochondria aren't functioning, you can't convert it to hormones. This is a primary reason hormone levels decline with chronic illness - it's not aging, it's mitochondrial shutdown.

These changes represent intelligent adaptation, not pathology. They're designed to help cells survive acute threats. But when the threat never resolves - when toxins continue accumulating, inflammation persists, infections smolder - the Cell Danger Response becomes chronic. Mitochondria remain locked in defensive mode, unable to return to normal function even when provided with all the nutrients and hormones they need.

The Mitochondria-Hormone Connection

The relationship between mitochondrial function and hormone health is not incidental - it's foundational. *Every aspect of hormone biology depends on adequate cellular energy.*

Hormone synthesis requires mitochondria. The conversion of cholesterol to pregnenolone - the first and rate-limiting step in all steroid hormone production - occurs exclusively in the inner mitochondrial membrane.[167] This includes cortisol, DHEA, testosterone, estrogen, and progesterone. When mitochondrial function is impaired, hormone production falls regardless of how much raw material is available or how much you try to stimulate the process.

Hormone receptors require energy. For a hormone to exert its effect, it must bind to a receptor, and that receptor must trigger intracellular signaling cascades. These processes are ATP-dependent.[47] When cellular energy is depleted, receptors become less responsive - not because the hormone isn't present, but because the cell lacks the energy to respond to it. This explains why patients can have optimal hormone levels yet experience all the symptoms of deficiency.

Hormone metabolism requires energy. The liver's processing of hormones - the conjugation reactions that prepare hormones for elimination - are energy-intensive processes.[168] When mitochondrial function fails, hormone metabolism slows, leading to accumulation of hormones and their metabolites. This contributes to estrogen dominance and the toxic metabolite buildup we discussed in earlier chapters.

Thyroid hormone activation requires energy. The conversion of T4 to active T3 is an ATP-dependent process.[169] Patients with mitochondrial dysfunction often show adequate T4 but low T3 - their bodies can't perform the conversion that activates thyroid hormone. Adding more T4 doesn't help because the conversion machinery isn't working.

This is why Lillian's hormone optimization strategy failed. Every hormone she took required mitochondrial energy to work - energy her cells weren't producing. Fixing the hormones without fixing the mitochondria was like adjusting the thermostat in a house with no electricity. The settings might be perfect, but nothing happens because there's no power to run the system.

T Phase Lifestyle Practices

The T Phase continues everything from previous phases while introducing practices that stimulate mitochondrial biogenesis - the creation of new mitochondria - and mitophagy - the clearing out of damaged ones.[170] These hormetic stressors - mild stressors that make your body stronger by triggering adaptive responses - must be carefully calibrated during mitochondrial recovery.

Progressive Exercise

Movement challenges your muscles to create more mitochondria to meet increased energy demands. But during mitochondrial recovery, too much too soon triggers Cell Danger Response while too little fails to stimulate adaptation. Start with gentle walking and progress to moderate aerobic activity as tolerance improves. Exercise should leave you feeling energized, not depleted. If you need more than 24 hours to recover from activity, you've exceeded your mitochondrial capacity - scale back and build more gradually.

Cold Exposure

Cold exposure activates brown fat and signals cells to produce more mitochondria for heat generation.[171] End your shower with 30 to 60 seconds of cold water, starting with cool water and gradually decreasing temperature over days and weeks as you adapt. Focus on breathing slowly and staying calm during the cold exposure - panicked breathing defeats the purpose by triggering stress responses. The key is consistency rather than intensity - daily brief cold exposure produces better results than occasional extreme cold.

Time-Restricted Eating

A 16:8 fasting pattern activates cellular cleanup processes including mitophagy - the selective destruction of damaged mitochondria.[147] Compress eating into an eight-hour window, fasting for sixteen hours overnight. This intermittent fasting trigger autophagy, allowing your cells to clear out dysfunctional mitochondria and make room for healthy new ones. Some patients need to ease into this gradually, starting with a 12-hour eating window and progressively narrowing over several weeks.

Heat Exposure

Sauna triggers heat shock proteins that support cellular repair and proper protein folding.[172] Use sauna three to four times per week for 15 to 20 minutes if available. Stay well hydrated and replace electrolytes lost through sweating. If sauna isn't available, hot baths provide similar though less intense benefits. The combination of heat and cold exposure creates a powerful hormetic signal for mitochondrial adaptation.

Senolytic Foods

Senescent cells are damaged cells that have stopped dividing but remain in tissues releasing inflammatory signals. Certain foods help clear them:[173] quercetin-rich foods like onions, apples, and berries; fisetin-rich foods especially strawberries; sulforaphane-rich foods like broccoli sprouts; and EGCG from green tea. Emphasize these foods in your meals throughout this phase.

T Phase Supplements

Once the terrain is prepared - drainage flowing, immune system balanced, toxins reduced - we can begin the delicate process of coaxing mitochondria back to full function. This isn't about forcing energy production through stimulation. It's about providing comprehensive support that addresses every aspect of mitochondrial biology. Follow your personalized MILA report for specific recommendations and dosing based on your assessment results.

Acetyl-L-Carnitine

This serves as the shuttle system that transports fatty acids into mitochondria for burning.[174] Without adequate carnitine, fats accumulate outside mitochondria while the engines inside starve for fuel. Beyond simple transport, it provides acetyl groups needed for the citric acid cycle and supports acetylcholine production for cognitive function. The acetyl form crosses the blood-brain barrier more efficiently than regular L-carnitine, supporting both physical energy and mental clarity.

Coenzyme Q10 (CoQ10)

CoQ10 is absolutely essential - it serves as the electron shuttle in the mitochondrial electron transport chain.[175] Without adequate CoQ10, the entire system backs up and electrons accumulate, generating damaging free radicals instead of ATP. The ubiquinol form is preferred over ubiquinone for those with chronic illness, as the conversion process may be impaired. CoQ10 also serves as a powerful antioxidant within mitochondrial membranes, protecting the very structures that produce energy.

B-Complex Vitamins

B vitamins serve as essential cofactors throughout energy metabolism.[176] B1 (thiamine) is required for pyruvate entry into the citric acid cycle - without it, glucose cannot be fully metabolized. B2 (riboflavin) forms FAD, a critical electron carrier. B3 (niacin) becomes NAD+, perhaps the most critical coenzyme in metabolism. B5 (pantothenic acid) forms coenzyme A, essential for the citric acid cycle.

The key is using activated, bioavailable forms at therapeutic doses adjusted for individual genetics - methylfolate instead of folic acid, methylcobalamin instead of cyanocobalamin. If you have MTHFR or other methylation variants, proper B vitamin selection is especially critical.

Magnesium

Magnesium is required for over 300 enzymatic reactions, but its role in mitochondrial function is particularly critical.[177] Every molecule of ATP must be bound to magnesium to be biologically active - it's actually Mg-ATP that cells use for energy. Without adequate magnesium, ATP cannot be utilized regardless of how much is produced.

Bioavailable forms include magnesium glycinate (calming, good for evening), magnesium malate (energizing, good for daytime), and magnesium threonate (crosses blood-brain barrier for cognitive support). Many patients benefit from using different forms at different times of day.

Continued Glutathione Support

Glutathione continues from previous phases, now serving critical mitochondrial protection.[178] Mitochondria maintain their own distinct glutathione pool, essential for neutralizing the reactive oxygen species inevitably generated during ATP production. Without adequate glutathione, increased mitochondrial activity generates oxidative stress that damages the very mitochondria we're trying to restore.

Practical Implementation: Your T Phase Protocol

The Turbocharge phase typically spans eight weeks. Here's what patients commonly experience:

Weeks 1-2: Subtle Awakening

Continue all previous phase practices. Transition to Turbocharge phase supplements as directed in your updated MILA report. Begin cold exposure with 30 seconds cool water at end of shower. Implement time-restricted eating with a 16:8 pattern. Initial improvements are often subtle - slightly better sleep quality, marginally improved morning energy, small increases in exercise tolerance. The mitochondria are beginning to respond but remain cautious.

Weeks 3-4: Momentum Builds

Increase cold exposure gradually to 45 to 60 seconds at colder temperature. Add sauna if available for 15 to 20 minutes, three times weekly. Progress exercise as tolerated. Energy improvements become more noticeable. Patients often report being able to do activities they couldn't tolerate before. For hormone patients, this is often when hormonal symptoms begin improving even without changing hormone doses.

Weeks 5-6: Breakthrough

For many patients, this is when the transformation becomes undeniable. Energy that felt forced or artificial in previous attempts now feels natural and sustainable. Sleep becomes more restorative. Physical capacity expands significantly. Mood stabilizes as neurotransmitter production normalizes with improved cellular energy. Hormone symptoms often improve dramatically as cells finally have the energy to respond to hormonal signals.

Weeks 7-8: Consolidation and Transition

Gains consolidate and stabilize. The mitochondria have established new patterns of function. Energy levels plateau at a significantly higher baseline than before the protocol. Complete MILA Progress Assessment to measure improvement and evaluate readiness for the Optimize phase.

When to Move Forward

You are ready to advance when you have completed eight weeks in the T Phase, your MILA Progress Assessment shows improvement, energy has meaningfully and sustainably improved, you are tolerating the supplements and hormetic practices well, and you can exercise without prolonged recovery. Energy should feel natural rather than forced or jittery.

Stay longer if energy improvements are minimal, if you continue to crash after activity, if brain fog persists significantly, or if you cannot tolerate the hormetic stressors without setbacks. Some patients with severe or long-standing mitochondrial dysfunction need additional weeks. The mitochondria are still rebuilding trust with their environment - don't rush the process.

Lillian's Transformation

Lillian completed the Eliminate and Strengthen phases before beginning Turbocharge - sixteen weeks of preparation that her previous practitioners had skipped entirely. They had jumped straight to hormone optimization without addressing the terrain that made hormone function possible.

Within two weeks of beginning the properly sequenced Turbocharge protocol, she noticed subtle improvements - she could walk to the mailbox without resting. By week four, she was walking around the block daily. By week eight, she had returned to teaching part-time and was beginning to consider light jogging again.

But the most remarkable change wasn't her energy - it was her hormones. Without changing any of her hormone medications, her symptoms had dramatically improved. The hot flashes that had persisted despite "optimal" estrogen levels had resolved. The mood swings that no amount of progesterone had touched had stabilized. The brain fog that thyroid optimization couldn't fix had lifted.

"My hormone levels are exactly the same as they were six months ago," Lillian said at her follow-up, reviewing her labs with amazement. "But I feel completely different. The hormones are finally working because my cells can finally use them."

Over the following months, we were actually able to reduce several of her hormone medications. As her mitochondria came back online, her body resumed producing more of its own hormones. The external support that had been necessary when her cells couldn't produce or respond to hormones became less necessary as cellular function restored.

"I spent three years trying to fix my hormones," Lillian reflected. "Six different practitioners, seventeen supplements, four prescriptions. And the answer wasn't in the hormones at all. The answer was in the mitochondria that make hormones work. Fix the engine, and the fuel finally does its job."

With mitochondrial function restored, the stage is set for the Optimize phase - where we address brain function, mood, and the neurological patterns that often persist even after physical energy returns. The brain, consuming 20 percent of the body's energy despite being only 2 percent of body weight, is exquisitely sensitive to mitochondrial function. Now that cellular energy production has been restored, we can address the complex neurological patterns that perpetuate illness and affect hormone signaling at the highest levels of regulation.

Key Takeaways

- Mitochondrial energy restoration must follow drainage optimization and immune rebalancing - attempting to force energy production while the terrain remains toxic and inflamed triggers Cell Danger Response and worsens symptoms rather than improving them.

- The Cell Danger Response is not mitochondrial failure but intelligent protection - mitochondria deliberately downshift into survival mode when they detect threats, reducing energy production while increasing hormone resistance, which explains why optimal hormone levels often produce no improvement in symptomatic patients.

- Hormone function depends entirely on mitochondrial function - steroid synthesis begins in mitochondria, hormone receptors require ATP to function, hormone metabolism requires cellular energy, and thyroid activation is ATP-dependent; fixing hormones without fixing mitochondria is futile.

- Lifestyle practices provide hormetic stress that stimulates mitochondrial biogenesis: progressive exercise challenges muscles to create more mitochondria, cold exposure activates brown fat, time-restricted eating triggers mitophagy, and heat exposure induces heat shock proteins.

- Effective mitochondrial supplementation requires comprehensive support: fuel transport through acetyl-L-carnitine, electron flow through CoQ10, metabolic catalysis through B-complex vitamins, energy utilization through magnesium, and antioxidant defense through continued glutathione.

- True hormonal vitality emerges not from hormone optimization alone but from creating conditions where mitochondria produce the energy that makes hormone synthesis and hormone response possible - working with the body's wisdom rather than trying to override it.

Chapter 16

O - Optimize

Restoring Brain and Nervous System Function

Warren was 55 years old and terrified he was developing early dementia. This former city planner had always prided himself on his sharp analytical mind - the ability to hold complex zoning regulations, environmental impact assessments, and community needs in his head simultaneously while crafting solutions that satisfied competing interests. Now he couldn't remember what he had eaten for breakfast.

"I lose words mid-sentence," Warren told me, his hands trembling slightly. "I'll be explaining something and suddenly the word I need just vanishes. Yesterday I forgot my own phone number - a number I've had for twenty years. I got lost driving to the grocery store I've been going to for a decade. My wife found the car keys in the refrigerator. I'm scared to death."

His cognitive decline had paralleled his hormonal decline over the past four years. His testosterone had dropped from a robust 680 to a concerning 285. His doctor started him on testosterone replacement, which helped his energy and libido but did nothing for his brain fog. Thyroid medication was added when his TSH crept up. Still no cognitive improvement. DHEA supplementation. Pregnenolone. A nootropic stack recommended by a biohacking podcast. Nothing touched the brain fog.

"My neurologist ran every test," Warren continued. "MRI, cognitive assessments, genetic testing for Alzheimer's risk. Everything came back normal. He said I'm just getting older, and this is what aging looks like. But I'm 55, not 85. My father was sharp as a tack until he died at 82. This isn't normal aging. Something is wrong."

He was right - it wasn't normal aging. His comprehensive history revealed the pattern. His cognitive decline had begun not with aging but with a period of severe chronic stress five years earlier - a contentious development project that had consumed eighteen months of 70-hour weeks, political battles, and public attacks on his professional judgment. He had never fully recovered from that period. Sleep became fragmented. Anxiety became his constant companion. And gradually, his sharp mind began to fade.

"Warren," I said, "your brain isn't failing because you're aging. Your brain is failing because your nervous system has been stuck in survival mode for five years. The chronic stress rewired your brain for danger detection rather than complex thinking. Your sleep disruption has prevented the glymphatic system from clearing metabolic waste from your brain. And the hormone treatments you've received - while addressing real deficiencies - haven't addressed the neurological patterns that are perpetuating the problem."

"You mean my brain fog isn't about my hormones?"

"Your hormones are part of it - testosterone and thyroid both affect cognitive function. But they're not the root cause. Your nervous system dysregulation is driving both your cognitive decline and your hormone imbalance. The hypothalamus - the brain region that controls hormone production - is also part of the stress response system. When your brain is stuck in survival mode, it changes how the hypothalamus signals hormone production. We need to optimize your brain function to optimize your hormones, not just the other way around."

The Intention of the Optimize Phase

The O Phase - Optimize - focuses on restoring brain and nervous system function. Its intention is to address the neurological patterns that persist even after drainage is established, immune function is balanced, and mitochondrial energy is restored. For many patients, this phase represents the completion of their healing journey - the point where cognitive clarity returns, mood stabilizes, and the nervous system finally shifts from chronic survival mode to normal function.[179]

The brain is the most energy-demanding organ in the body, consuming approximately 20 percent of total metabolic output despite comprising only 2 percent of body weight.[180] This extraordinary metabolic demand makes the brain exquisitely sensitive to everything we've addressed in previous phases - toxic burden, immune dysregulation, and mitochondrial dysfunction. But the brain also has unique vulnerabilities and requirements that merit dedicated attention.

For hormone patients, the Optimize phase holds special significance. The hypothalamus - the master regulator of hormonal function - is a brain structure. The pituitary gland receives its instructions from the brain. Neurotransmitters and hormones share biosynthetic pathways and intimately influence each other. You cannot fully optimize hormones without optimizing the brain that controls them.

The Brain-Hormone Axis

The relationship between brain function and hormone balance is bidirectional and profound. Hormones affect brain function, and brain function affects hormone production. Understanding this relationship explains why Warren's hormone treatments failed to restore his cognition - and why optimizing brain function is essential for lasting hormone balance.

The hypothalamus controls hormone production. This small brain structure at the base of the brain serves as the master regulator of the entire endocrine system.[12] It releases hormones that tell the pituitary what to do, and the pituitary then signals the thyroid, adrenals, and gonads. When the hypothalamus is dysregulated - whether from stress, inflammation, or toxicity - the entire hormonal cascade is affected. No amount of downstream hormone replacement fully corrects hypothalamic dysfunction.

Chronic stress rewires the hypothalamus. Prolonged activation of the stress response literally changes hypothalamic structure and function.[25] The hypothalamus becomes hypersensitive to threat signals and less responsive to feedback that should turn off the stress response. This creates the pattern Warren experienced - a brain stuck in survival mode that keeps signaling for stress hormones while suppressing reproductive and thyroid hormones.

Neurotransmitters and hormones share precursors. The amino acid tyrosine is converted into both dopamine and thyroid hormone. Tryptophan becomes both serotonin and melatonin.[111] When neurotransmitter production is impaired, hormone production suffers - and vice versa. The brain fog, mood changes, and cognitive decline that hormone patients experience often reflect neurotransmitter imbalances as much as hormone imbalances.

Hormones are neuroprotective. Estrogen, progesterone, testosterone, and thyroid hormone all have direct effects on brain cells. They support neuroplasticity, protect against oxidative damage, maintain myelin, and influence neurotransmitter production.[28] When these hormones decline - whether from aging, stress, or illness - brain function suffers. But simply replacing hormones often isn't enough if the brain itself is dysregulated.

The Glymphatic System: Your Brain's Drainage Network

One of the most significant neuroscience discoveries of the past decade is the glymphatic system - the brain's dedicated waste clearance network.[181] Unlike the rest of the body, the brain has no lymphatic vessels. Instead, it relies on a specialized system that uses cerebrospinal fluid to flush metabolic waste from brain tissue.

This system operates primarily during deep sleep. During waking hours, the spaces between brain cells are narrow, limiting fluid flow. During deep sleep, these spaces expand by up to 60 percent, allowing cerebrospinal fluid to flow through and carry away accumulated waste - including beta-amyloid protein associated with Alzheimer's disease.[182]

When sleep is disrupted - as it commonly is in chronic illness, chronic stress, and hormone imbalance - glymphatic function suffers. Metabolic waste accumulates in brain tissue. Inflammation increases. Cognitive function declines. This explains why sleep disruption so powerfully affects brain fog and cognitive function - it's not just about rest, it's about waste clearance.

Warren's sleep had been fragmented for five years - rarely achieving more than four consecutive hours of sleep. His glymphatic system had been compromised for years, allowing metabolic waste to accumulate in his brain tissue. No hormone treatment could compensate for this fundamental drainage failure.

The Vagus Nerve: The Rest-and-Digest Highway

The vagus nerve is the longest cranial nerve in the body, connecting the brainstem to virtually every major organ - heart, lungs, digestive tract, liver, spleen, and kidneys. It serves as the primary pathway of the parasympathetic nervous system - the "rest and digest" branch that opposes the sympathetic "fight or flight" response.[183]

Vagal tone - the strength and responsiveness of vagus nerve signaling - determines how quickly you can shift from stress response to relaxation response. High vagal tone means rapid recovery from stress. Low vagal tone means getting stuck in stress response, unable to return to baseline even when the threat has passed.

Chronic stress, trauma, and chronic illness all reduce vagal tone.[109] The vagus nerve becomes less responsive, making it increasingly difficult to activate the parasympathetic state needed for healing, digestion, hormone production, and cognitive function. This is why chronically stressed individuals often have digestive problems, hormone imbalances, and difficulty thinking clearly - their vagus nerve can't activate the rest-and-digest state needed for these functions.

For hormone health specifically, vagal tone directly affects the hypothalamic-pituitary axis. The parasympathetic state is required for normal hormone production signaling. When vagal tone is low and the body is stuck in sympathetic overdrive, the hypothalamus prioritizes stress hormone production over reproductive and thyroid hormones - the physiological basis of pregnenolone steal we discussed earlier.

O Phase Lifestyle Practices

The Optimize phase continues everything from previous phases while adding specific practices to restore vagal tone, support glymphatic function, and rebuild healthy neurological patterns.

Sleep Optimization

Sleep is non-negotiable for brain restoration. The glymphatic system requires deep sleep to function. Target seven to nine hours nightly with consistent bed and wake times.[184] Create a cool, completely dark sleep environment. Avoid screens for at least one hour before bed - blue light suppresses melatonin production. Consider sleep tracking to identify patterns and disruptions.

Sleep position affects glymphatic drainage - side sleeping, particularly on the right side, enhances cerebrospinal fluid flow compared to back or stomach sleeping.[185] If you've been a back sleeper, transitioning to side sleeping may improve brain waste clearance.

Vagal Toning Exercises

The vagus nerve can be strengthened like a muscle through specific practices:[186]

Cold exposure: Brief cold exposure activates the vagus nerve. Continue the cold shower practice from the Turbocharge phase, focusing on slow, controlled breathing during the cold exposure.

Gargling: Vigorous gargling activates the vagus nerve branches that innervate the throat. Gargle water forcefully for 30 to 60 seconds, several times daily, until your eyes water slightly.

Humming and chanting: Vocal vibrations stimulate the vagus nerve. Humming, singing, or chanting "Om" for several minutes activates parasympathetic pathways.

Deep breathing: Continue the MILA breathing technique. Extended exhales particularly activate the vagus nerve - inhale for 4 counts, exhale for 8 counts.

Cognitive Engagement

The brain requires stimulation to maintain function and build new neural connections.[187] Engage in activities that challenge your brain - learning new skills, reading challenging material, strategic games, musical instruments, new languages. The key is novelty and challenge - activities that push beyond your current abilities stimulate neuroplasticity more than familiar activities performed on autopilot.

Nature Exposure

Time in natural environments reduces cortisol, activates the parasympathetic nervous system, and improves cognitive function.[188] Aim for at least 20 minutes daily in natural settings - parks, forests, gardens, or any green space. If outdoor access is limited, even viewing nature images or keeping plants indoors provides some benefit, though less than actual nature immersion.

Social Connection

The vagus nerve is activated by positive social interaction.[189] Eye contact, conversation, physical touch, and a sense of belonging all signal safety to the nervous system, promoting parasympathetic activation. Isolation and loneliness do the opposite - they signal threat and maintain sympathetic overdrive. Prioritize meaningful social connection as a neurological intervention, not just emotional support.

O Phase Supplements

The O Phase supplements support sleep quality, brain function, and neurotransmitter balance. With the foundational phases complete, the brain can finally utilize these supports effectively. Follow your personalized MILA report for specific recommendations and dosing based on your assessment results.

Sleep Support Formula

This supplement promotes relaxation and healthy neurotransmitter balance for falling asleep and achieving restorative sleep stages. It supports the transition from waking consciousness to deep sleep where glymphatic clearance occurs. Unlike pharmaceutical sleep aids that provide sedation without true restoration, this formula supports natural sleep architecture. Take as directed in the evening, typically 30 to 60 minutes before bed.

Magnesium Threonate

This specialized form of magnesium crosses the blood-brain barrier effectively to support brain magnesium levels.[190] Once in the brain, magnesium enhances GABA receptor sensitivity, amplifying GABA's calming effects. GABA is the brain's primary inhibitory neurotransmitter - it slows neural activity, reduces anxiety, and creates the calm that allows sleep. When GABA function is low, the brain can't downshift. Racing thoughts continue even when you want to sleep.

Studies show magnesium threonate improves cognitive function, memory, and sleep quality. Unlike other magnesium forms that primarily affect the body, threonate specifically targets neural tissue. It's particularly valuable for patients with significant brain fog, anxiety, or sleep difficulties.

Neurological Support Remedy

This supplement enhances glymphatic drainage and brain circulation, supporting the brain's waste clearance systems. It helps optimize the fluid dynamics that allow cerebrospinal fluid to wash through neural tissue during sleep, carrying away the metabolic debris that contributes to brain fog and cognitive impairment. It also supports healthy blood flow to the brain, ensuring adequate delivery of oxygen and nutrients to neural tissue.

Continued Glutathione Support

Glutathione continues throughout this phase for brain protection during increased neural activity and repair. The brain requires enormous quantities of glutathione to manage the oxidative stress generated by its intensive metabolic activity.[191] As neuroplasticity increases during the O Phase - as the brain actively rewires and repairs - antioxidant protection becomes even more critical.

Without adequate glutathione, the increased neural activity of recovery would generate oxidative damage faster than repair could address. Continue liposomal or S-acetyl glutathione as in previous phases.

Practical Implementation: Your O Phase Protocol

The Optimize phase typically spans six to eight weeks. Here's what patients commonly experience:

Weeks 1-2: Sleep Foundation

Continue all previous phase practices. Transition to Optimize phase supplements as directed in your updated MILA report. Implement strict sleep hygiene - consistent timing, dark room, no screens one to two hours before bed, no alcohol. Begin the MILA deep breathing practice twice daily. Initial improvements often appear in sleep quality - falling asleep faster, fewer awakenings, feeling slightly more refreshed upon waking.

Weeks 3-4: Cognitive Clearing

Brain fog typically begins lifting during this period. Word-finding improves. Mental processing speeds up. Patients often describe it as "the lights coming back on" - subtle at first, then increasingly noticeable. Mood often stabilizes as neurotransmitter production normalizes. Anxiety, particularly evening anxiety, tends to decrease.

Weeks 5-6: Mental Clarity Returns

For many patients, this is when cognitive function feels genuinely restored. Complex thinking becomes easier. Memory improves - both forming new memories and accessing old ones. Creativity returns. The experience of being fully present that had been missing becomes available again. Sleep becomes deeply restorative.

Weeks 7-8: Consolidation and Integration

Gains consolidate and stabilize. The brain has established new patterns of function. Cognitive capacity plateaus at a significantly higher baseline. Emotional regulation feels natural rather than effortful. Complete MILA Progress Assessment to measure improvement and evaluate readiness for the final phases.

When to Move Forward

You are ready to advance when you have completed six to eight weeks in the O Phase and your MILA Progress Assessment shows improvement. Within the assessment should show brain fog has meaningfully lifted, sleep is restorative, mood is stable, and you can think clearly and access words without difficulty. Cognitive function should feel natural rather than requiring constant effort.

Stay longer if brain fog persists significantly, if sleep remains unrestorative despite good sleep hygiene, if mood instability continues, or if cognitive function has not meaningfully improved. Some patients with long-standing neurological symptoms, significant blood-brain barrier damage, or history of head injury need additional weeks. The brain is rebuilding complex neural networks - don't rush the process.

Warren's Transformation

Warren completed the full R.E.S.T.O.R.E. sequence before reaching the Optimize phase - nearly five months of systematic terrain restoration. By the time he began the brain-focused interventions, his drainage was flowing, his immune system was balanced, and his mitochondria were producing energy. But his brain fog had persisted, and his fear of dementia remained.

The sleep optimization was transformative. After five years of fragmented sleep, achieving seven consecutive hours felt miraculous. "I forgot what it felt like to actually wake up rested," he said at his four-week follow-up. "My wife says I'm a different person in the morning."

The vagal toning exercises - which he initially found odd - produced noticeable effects within two weeks. His chronic anxiety began to ease. The constant sense of being on edge that had been his companion for five years started to lift. He could feel his nervous system shifting from survival mode to something closer to normal.

By week six, the cognitive breakthrough arrived. "I was in a meeting yesterday," Warren recounted, his eyes bright for the first time since I'd met him, "and I realized I was tracking five different stakeholder perspectives simultaneously, synthesizing them into a solution, and presenting it coherently - all without struggling. That's the old me. That's who I used to be before all this started."

His word-finding difficulties had resolved. His memory had returned. The car keys stayed out of the refrigerator. He could remember what he had eaten for breakfast and dinner the night before. Along with the complex details of the project, he was working on.

"I was so afraid I was losing my mind," Warren reflected at his final Optimize phase assessment. "Turns out my mind was fine - it was just stuck in survival mode, unable to do the complex thinking it was designed for because it was too busy scanning for threats. My brain wasn't failing from age. It was failing from unrelenting stress that had never resolved. Once we gave it the conditions it needed - proper sleep, calm nervous system, right nutrients - it came back online. I'm not developing dementia. I was developing a nervous system that forgot how to rest."

With brain function restored and nervous system regulation achieved, the final phases of the R.E.S.T.O.R.E. MILA protocol address what comes after acute restoration - the Repair phase for structural healing and the Everlasting phase for sustainable maintenance. These phases acknowledge that true healing isn't complete when symptoms are resolved. The body requires time to fully repair damaged tissues, and lasting wellness requires ongoing practices that maintain the gains achieved throughout the protocol. In the next chapter, we explore how to consolidate your healing and create the foundation for lifelong hormonal health.

Key Takeaways

- The brain controls hormone production through the hypothalamus-pituitary axis; chronic stress rewires the hypothalamus to prioritize survival hormones over reproductive and thyroid hormones, creating hormone imbalances that cannot be fully corrected without addressing the underlying neurological dysregulation.

- The glymphatic system - the brain's dedicated waste clearance network - operates primarily during deep sleep; disrupted sleep prevents metabolic waste clearance from brain tissue, contributing to brain fog, cognitive decline, and neuroinflammation regardless of hormone optimization.

- Vagal tone determines how quickly you can shift from stress response to relaxation; low vagal tone keeps the nervous system stuck in sympathetic overdrive, impairing digestion, hormone production, and cognitive function while perpetuating the stress that caused the problem.

- Specific practices restore vagal tone and nervous system balance: cold exposure, gargling, humming, extended exhale breathing, nature exposure, and positive social connection all activate the parasympathetic pathways needed for healing and hormone regulation.

- The O Phase supplements support sleep and brain function: sleep support formula for natural sleep architecture, magnesium threonate for brain-specific magnesium delivery, neurological support remedy for glymphatic drainage, and continued glutathione for antioxidant protection during neural repair.

- The O Phase typically produces the cognitive breakthrough that hormone patients have been seeking - brain fog lifts, memory returns, and the nervous system finally shifts from survival mode to normal function, allowing proper hypothalamic regulation of hormonal production.

Chapter 17

R and E - Repair and Everlasting

Consolidating Healing and Maintaining Wellness

Iris was sitting in my office for her six-month follow-up, and I almost didn't recognize her. This 59-year-old retired elementary school teacher had arrived at my practice eight months earlier looking at least a decade older than her age - exhausted, puffy, moving slowly, her eyes dull with the fatigue of someone who had been fighting her own body for too long.

Now she radiated vitality. Her skin had a healthy glow. Her eyes were bright and engaged. She moved with energy and purpose. She had lost twenty-five pounds of inflammatory weight without trying. Her chronic joint pain had resolved. Her brain fog had lifted. Her hot flashes and night sweats - which had plagued her for seven years despite multiple hormone interventions - were gone.

"I feel like myself again," Iris said, tears welling in her eyes. "For seven years, I forgot who I was. I thought this was just what getting older meant - being tired all the time, hurting everywhere, not being able to think clearly, gaining weight no matter what I did. I thought I had to accept it. But this isn't aging. This is what happens when your body finally works the way it's supposed to."

Her transformation had followed the complete R.E.S.T.O.R.E. MILA sequence over seven months. The Eliminate phase had opened her drainage pathways and removed the toxic burden overwhelming her liver's ability to metabolize hormones. The Strengthen phase had calmed her immune system's chronic inflammatory state. The Turbocharge phase had restored the mitochondrial function that made hormone production and response possible. The Optimize phase had rebalanced her nervous system and restored her cognitive function.

"So, what now?" Iris asked the question that brought her to this appointment. "I feel amazing. But I'm terrified of going backward. I've worked so hard to get here. How do I make sure I don't lose everything I've gained?"

It was the right question - and the reason the R.E.S.T.O.R.E. protocol doesn't end with Optimize. "Iris," I said, "the last two letters of the protocol - R and E, Repair and Everlasting - are about exactly that. Repair addresses the structural healing that continues after symptoms resolve. Everlasting creates sustainable practices that maintain your gains for life. You've done the hard work of acute restoration. Now we consolidate that healing and build the foundation for permanent wellness."

The Intention of Repair and Everlasting

The final phases of the R.E.S.T.O.R.E. MILA protocol acknowledge a truth that most healing programs ignore: feeling better is not the same as being healed. Symptoms can resolve while underlying tissue damage remains. Energy can return while cellular repair continues. Hormones can balance while the systems that maintain them remain fragile.[99]

The Repair phase focuses on structural healing - supporting the body's ongoing work of tissue regeneration, cellular renewal, and system consolidation. The Everlasting phase establishes the sustainable practices, minimal supplementation, and body awareness that maintain wellness for life.

Together, these phases prevent the relapse that plagues so many patients who improve temporarily only to slide back into illness. They transform acute recovery into lasting transformation.

The Repair Phase: Structural Healing

Your body is constantly rebuilding itself. Red blood cells are replaced every 120 days. Your gut lining regenerates every 3 to 5 days. Bone is completely remodeled every 10 years.[192] This continuous regeneration means that the body you have today is literally not the same body you had a year ago - it has been rebuilt, cell by cell, tissue by tissue.

During chronic illness, this regeneration process is compromised. Damaged cells are replaced with more damaged cells. Tissues are rebuilt with inferior materials. The body copies its dysfunction rather than correcting it. This is why chronic illness perpetuates - the body keeps rebuilding itself in its broken state.

The Repair phase supports the transition from building a broken body to building a healthy one. With drainage established, immune function balanced, mitochondrial energy restored, and nervous system regulated, your body can finally rebuild properly. But this rebuilding takes time - and it benefits from continued support.[29]

For hormone patients specifically, the Repair phase allows hormone-producing tissues to regenerate. Ovarian cells that were damaged by autoimmune attack can be replaced. Thyroid tissue that was inflamed can heal. Adrenal glands that were exhausted can rebuild. This structural repair is what separates temporary symptom improvement from lasting hormone restoration.

Repair Phase Practices

The Repair phase continues all foundational practices from previous phases while emphasizing factors that support tissue regeneration.

Continued Dietary Excellence

The Toxic Nine remain permanently eliminated - this is non-negotiable for long-term health. Focus on nutrient density: organ meats, bone broth, colorful vegetables, wild-caught fish, pastured eggs. These foods provide the raw materials - amino acids, minerals, fatty acids - that your body needs to rebuild healthy tissue. Collagen-rich foods like bone broth specifically support connective tissue repair throughout the body.

Protein Optimization

Tissue repair requires adequate protein - more than most people consume, especially as they age.[193] Aim for 0.7 to 1 gram of protein per pound of body weight daily, distributed across meals. This provides the amino acids needed for cellular repair, enzyme production, and hormone synthesis. Many patients find their tissue healing accelerates when protein intake is optimized.

Sleep Prioritization

Growth hormone - critical for tissue repair - is released primarily during deep sleep. The Repair phase demands even more attention to sleep quality than previous phases. Seven to nine hours nightly, consistent timing, dark and cool environment, and minimal evening stimulation. Sleep is when your body does its rebuilding work - shortchanging sleep shortchanges repair.

Stress Management

Chronic stress diverts resources from repair to survival.[194] Continue all vagal toning practices from the Optimize phase. Add whatever stress management techniques resonate with you - meditation, yoga, time in nature, creative pursuits, meaningful social connection. The parasympathetic state is the repair state; you cannot fully heal while stuck in sympathetic overdrive.

Appropriate Movement

Movement stimulates tissue repair through mechanical signaling, improved circulation, and growth factor release.[195] By the Repair phase, most patients can engage in moderate exercise without setbacks. Build toward a sustainable routine that includes resistance training for muscle and bone, cardiovascular work for heart and circulation, and flexibility work for connective tissue. Exercise should energize, not deplete.

R-E Phase Supplements: The Minimal Effective Dose

One of the most common questions I receive from patients completing the protocol is: "How many supplements do I need to take forever?" The question reveals a fundamental misunderstanding about what true healing means. If you need dozens of supplements indefinitely to maintain wellness, you haven't actually restored terrain - you've just found a more sophisticated way to manage symptoms.

Real healing reduces dependency, not increases it. By the time you reach these final phases, most patients find they can maintain vibrant wellness with a surprisingly minimal regimen. Follow your personalized MILA report for specific recommendations based on your assessment results.

Foundation Multivitamin

A high-quality multivitamin provides foundational nutrients in bioavailable forms, covering common dietary gaps without mega-dosing individual nutrients.[196]

Omega-3 Fatty Acids

Continue omega-3 supplementation to maintain cellular membrane integrity and support the production of specialized pro-resolving mediators that keep inflammation balanced.[54] This is one supplement that provides ongoing benefit for virtually everyone.

Vitamin D3 with K2

These nutrients support immune regulation, bone health, and countless other functions. Target optimal ranges of 50 to 70 ng/mL for vitamin D, not just "normal" ranges.[197]

Structural Support (R Phase)

For patients with specific structural repair needs identified through Dynamic Intake assessment, targeted collagen peptides and minerals may be indicated temporarily. Collagen provides the raw materials for connective tissue synthesis but must be dosed appropriately - typically 10 to 20 grams daily - so the body can utilize it without overwhelming lymphatic clearance capacity. Antioxidants like NAC and CoQ10 protect tissues during active repair.

That's it for most people. Four to five supplements. Not forty. Not the shopping bag of bottles that many patients arrive with initially. Because when terrain is restored, the body maintains balance naturally.

Body Literacy: Recognizing Early Signals

Perhaps the most valuable skill developed through the R.E.S.T.O.R.E. MILA protocol is body literacy - the ability to recognize your body's early warning signals and respond before small issues become big problems.[198]

Your body constantly communicates its state. Chronic illness often develops because we've learned to ignore or override these signals. The Everlasting phase cultivates deep attention to the subtle messages your body sends:

Energy patterns: Notice when your energy dips. Is it after certain foods? Activities? Times of day? These patterns reveal what supports and what depletes you.

Sleep quality: Pay attention to sleep onset, middle-of-night waking, dream patterns, and morning energy. Sleep changes are often early indicators of emerging imbalances.

Digestive function: Monitor bowel regularity, bloating, food reactions. Digestive changes often precede systemic symptoms by weeks or months.

Mood and cognition: Notice irritability, anxiety, brain fog, difficulty concentrating. These may signal hormonal shifts, blood sugar issues, or inflammatory triggers before physical symptoms appear.

Physical signs: Watch for skin changes, puffiness, joint stiffness, temperature intolerance. These visible signals often reflect internal changes that can be addressed early.

Seasonal Resets

Even with excellent maintenance, most bodies benefit from periodic intensive support. The Everlasting phase incorporates quarterly or seasonal "resets" - brief returns to more therapeutic protocols that prevent accumulated imbalances from developing into problems.

A seasonal reset might include a week of stricter dietary adherence - eliminating any foods that have crept back in. It might involve returning to drainage support for a few weeks to clear any accumulation. It might include a brief period of enhanced antioxidant support or a focused detoxification protocol.[199]

Think of seasonal resets as preventive maintenance - changing the oil before the engine shows signs of trouble. The investment of a few weeks of enhanced support quarterly can prevent the months of intensive work required to recover from a significant relapse.

When to Seek Support

Body literacy includes recognizing when you need help. The Everlasting phase doesn't mean going at it alone - it means maintaining awareness that allows early intervention when needed.

Consider returning to more intensive support if symptoms that had resolved begin returning, if you experience a significant stressor - illness, trauma, major life change, if blood work shows markers trending in concerning directions, if seasonal resets aren't producing their usual benefits, or if you simply feel that something is "off" even without specific symptoms. Early intervention prevents small imbalances from becoming major setbacks.

Iris's Ongoing Journey

At her twelve-month follow-up - six months into the Everlasting phase - Iris was thriving. Her supplement protocol had simplified to omega-3s, a foundation multivitamin, and vitamin D3 with K2. Her dietary practices had become second nature - the Toxic Nine foods held no appeal because she knew how they made her feel. Her exercise routine was consistent and enjoyable. Her sleep was restorative.

"I had a moment last month," Iris shared. "I was at my granddaughter's birthday party, surrounded by cake and pizza, feeling energetic and clear-headed while everyone around me was in food comas. And I realized - this is my new normal. I'm not depriving myself. I'm just choosing to feel good."

She had experienced one minor setback - a stressful family situation had triggered a few weeks of sleep disruption and returning fatigue. But she recognized the pattern early, returned briefly to enhanced drainage and nervous system support, and recovered quickly. "Before, that stress would have sent me into a month-long spiral," she said. "Now I have tools. I know what to do. I caught it early and addressed it before it became a problem."

Her hormone levels - which had been chaotic for seven years before the protocol - had stabilized without any hormone replacement. Her estrogen and progesterone fluctuated naturally with her cycle. Her thyroid function had normalized. Her adrenal output had balanced. The hormones that had been "imbalanced" were never actually the problem - they were symptoms of a terrain that couldn't support proper hormone function. Once the terrain was restored, the hormones followed.

"I used to think hormone balance was about finding the right pill or cream or supplement," Iris reflected. "Now I understand that hormone balance is about creating a body that can make and use hormones properly. The terrain determines the hormones, not the other way around. Fix the terrain, and the hormones take care of themselves."

Iris's journey - from exhausted, puffy, cognitively impaired, and hormonally chaotic to vibrant, clear-minded, and naturally balanced - illustrates the core message of this entire book. Hormone imbalance is not a cause; it is a symptom. The endless adjustment of hormone levels that characterizes conventional and functional medicine approaches treats the symptom while ignoring the cause. True restoration requires addressing the terrain - the mitochondrial function, immune balance, lymphatic flow, and nervous system regulation that determines whether hormones are produced, metabolized, and responded to properly. In our concluding chapter, we'll synthesize everything we've explored and chart the path forward for your own hormonal restoration.

Key Takeaways

- Feeling better is not the same as being healed - the Repair phase supports ongoing tissue regeneration and structural healing that continues after symptoms resolve, giving hormone-producing tissues time to fully regenerate rather than stopping treatment when you merely feel improved.

- The Repair phase emphasizes factors that support tissue regeneration: continued dietary excellence with the Toxic Nine permanently eliminated, optimized protein intake for cellular repair, prioritized sleep for growth hormone release, stress management for parasympathetic repair states, and appropriate movement for mechanical signaling.

- Real healing reduces dependency - most patients maintain vibrant wellness with just four to five supplements: a foundation multivitamin, omega-3 fatty acids, vitamin D3 with

K2, and temporary structural support if needed, not the dozens of supplements that characterize symptom management approaches.

- Body literacy - the ability to recognize early warning signals and respond before small issues become big problems - is the most valuable skill developed through the protocol; chronic illness often develops because we've learned to ignore or override these signals.

- Seasonal resets - quarterly returns to more intensive support - prevent accumulated imbalances from developing into problems, serving as preventive maintenance that avoids the extensive work required to recover from significant relapse.

- The terrain determines the hormones - when the body can properly produce, metabolize, and respond to hormones because drainage flows, immunity balances, mitochondria function, and the nervous system regulates, hormone levels often stabilize without direct hormone intervention.

Conclusion

The Path Forward

We began this book with a simple but revolutionary premise: hormone imbalance is a symptom, not a cause. Throughout these pages, we've explored why this matters - why understanding hormones as downstream manifestations of deeper dysfunction changes everything about how we approach hormonal health.

You've met patients whose stories likely resonate with your own experience. Margaret, who spent years adjusting hormone doses while the underlying dysfunction remained unaddressed. Maureen, who chased hormone imbalances for four years before discovering that her MILA dysfunction was the true problem. Rosemary, whose estrogen dominance resolved not through hormone adjustment but through opening her drainage pathways. Claire, whose Hashimoto's improved dramatically when she stopped eliminating foods unnecessarily and started nourishing her terrain properly. Janelle, whose autoimmune attack on her ovaries slowed when her immune system learned to regulate itself again. Lillian, whose "optimal" hormone levels produced no benefit until her mitochondria came back online. Warren, whose cognitive decline reversed when his brain emerged from survival mode. And Iris, whose complete transformation demonstrated what becomes possible when the full terrain is addressed.

Each of these patients had been failed by the same approach - the approach that dominates both conventional and functional medicine. Their hormones were tested, found abnormal, and treated. When treatment failed or produced only temporary improvement, doses were adjusted, hormones were added, protocols were intensified. The assumption was always that hormones were the problem and hormone manipulation was the solution.

That assumption is wrong. And continuing to operate from that assumption is why millions of people remain trapped in hormonal dysfunction despite endless interventions.

The Paradigm Shift

The shift from treating hormones as the cause to understanding them as symptoms requires a fundamental reorientation - a paradigm shift in how we think about the body and health.

The old paradigm says: Your hormones are imbalanced. Let's measure them, identify the deficiencies or excesses, and correct them with replacement or suppression. When that doesn't work, let's adjust the doses, try different forms, add more hormones to the mix. The body is a machine with broken parts that need fixing.

The new paradigm says: Your hormones are imbalanced because something is wrong with the terrain that produces, metabolizes, and responds to them. Let's identify and address that underlying dysfunction - the mitochondrial shutdown, the immune dysregulation, the lymphatic congestion, the nervous system imbalance - and watch the hormones often normalize on their own. The body is an intelligent, self-regulating system that produces symptoms for good reasons.

This shift doesn't mean hormones never need treatment. Some patients require hormone support while their terrain heals. Some have permanent damage to hormone-producing organs that necessitates lifelong replacement. But even in these cases, addressing the terrain determines how effectively hormone support works - whether the cells can actually respond to the hormones provided, whether the liver can metabolize them properly, whether the immune system will attack the organs receiving them.

The MILA Framework

The Mitochondrial-Immune-Lymphatic Axis provides the framework for understanding terrain dysfunction and addressing it systematically.

Mitochondria are where hormone synthesis begins. The conversion of cholesterol to pregnenolone - the first step in producing all steroid hormones - happens inside the mitochondria. When mitochondrial function is impaired, hormone production fails regardless of how much raw material is available. And when the Cell Danger Response locks mitochondria in survival mode, cells become resistant to hormones even when levels are optimal.

Immune function shapes hormone health in ways both obvious and subtle. Autoimmune attacks directly destroy hormone-producing tissues - the thyroid in Hashimoto's, the ovaries in autoimmune oophoritis, the adrenals in Addison's disease. Chronic inflammation drives aromatase activity, triggers pregnenolone steal, and impairs thyroid conversion. The immune system and endocrine system are not separate - they're intimately connected.

Lymphatic flow determines whether hormones are properly cleared after they've done their work. When lymphatic drainage is impaired, hormone metabolites accumulate. The liver's conjugated estrogens can't reach the gut for elimination. Estrogen dominance often reflects not excessive production, but inadequate clearance - a drainage problem rather than a production problem.

These three systems - mitochondrial, immune, and lymphatic - are not independent. They form an interconnected axis where dysfunction in one drives dysfunction in the others. Mitochondrial failure impairs immune cell function. Immune dysregulation damages mitochondria. Lymphatic stagnation allows both toxins and inflammatory mediators to accumulate, worsening both mitochondrial and immune function. This interconnection is why isolated interventions often fail and why systematic restoration through the R.E.S.T.O.R.E. MILA protocol produces results that individual treatments cannot achieve.

The R.E.S.T.O.R.E. Sequence

The R.E.S.T.O.R.E. MILA protocol provides a systematic approach to terrain restoration that makes lasting hormone balance possible.

Reveal uncovers the specific patterns of dysfunction driving your symptoms. Through the Dynamic Intake and Fundamental Four testing, you identify not just what's wrong but why - the upstream causes that create downstream hormone imbalances.

Eliminate opens drainage pathways and removes the toxic burden overwhelming your system. You cannot detoxify while continuing to pour toxins in, and you cannot mobilize stored toxins while drainage pathways are blocked. This phase establishes the foundation everything else builds upon.

Strengthen restores immune intelligence - teaching your immune system to regulate itself rather than remain stuck in chronic activation or attacking your own tissues. For hormone patients, this phase is critical because immune dysregulation directly drives hormonal dysfunction.

Turbocharge brings mitochondria back online - restoring the cellular energy production that makes hormone synthesis, hormone response, and hormone metabolism possible. This phase can only succeed after drainage is open and immune function is balanced.

Optimize addresses brain and nervous system function - rebalancing the neurological patterns that control hormone production through the hypothalamic-pituitary axis and affect every aspect of health and healing.

Repair supports ongoing tissue regeneration after symptoms resolve - giving hormone-producing organs time to fully heal rather than stopping treatment when you merely feel better.

Everlasting establishes the sustainable practices that maintain your gains for life - minimal supplementation, body literacy, and the ongoing awareness that prevents small imbalances from becoming major problems.

This sequence is not arbitrary. Each phase builds on the previous ones, creating conditions that make the next phase possible. Attempting to skip phases or reverse the order typically produces temporary improvement followed by relapse - as countless patients have experienced when practitioners jumped straight to mitochondrial support or hormone optimization without first addressing drainage and immune function.

Your Next Steps

If you recognize yourself in these pages - if you've been chasing hormone imbalances without lasting success, if you've been told your labs are normal while you feel terrible, if you've been adding hormone after hormone without achieving the vitality you seek - the path forward begins with a single step.

Visit restoremila.com and complete the Dynamic Intake. This intelligent assessment will reveal the patterns of dysfunction underlying your symptoms and generate your personalized MILA report with specific recommendations for beginning your restoration journey. While there is a small administrative fee to maintain the system, this fee is fully reimbursed with your first purchase.

The Dynamic Intake doesn't replace working with a qualified practitioner - and for complex cases, professional guidance is invaluable. But it provides something most practitioners don't offer: a systematic framework for understanding your unique pattern of dysfunction and a clear sequence for addressing it.

If you're working with a practitioner, share this book with them. The R.E.S.T.O.R.E. MILA framework can complement their approach, providing structure and sequencing that enhances whatever modalities they use. Most practitioners genuinely want to help their patients - they've simply been trained in the hormone-as-cause paradigm and may not have been exposed to the terrain-based approach.

A Final Word on Hope

If you've been struggling with hormonal dysfunction for months or years, you may have lost hope. You may have been told that this is just what aging looks like, that you'll have to manage these symptoms for the rest of your life, that there's nothing more that can be done. You may have internalized the message that your body has failed you and that hormone replacement is your only option.

I want to offer you a different message: *Your body hasn't failed you. It's been communicating with you all along through symptoms that signal underlying dysfunction.* Those symptoms aren't random - they're intelligent responses to real problems. And those problems can be addressed.

The patients in this book - Margaret, Maureen, Rosemary, Claire, Janelle, Lillian, Warren, Iris, and all the others - had lost hope too. They had tried everything conventional and functional medicine offered. They had been told their conditions were permanent, their symptoms inevitable, their options exhausted. And yet they recovered. Not through finding the right hormone formula, but through addressing the terrain that made hormone function possible.

Your body wants to heal. It's designed to heal. Given the right conditions - drainage flowing, immune system balanced, mitochondria functioning, nervous system regulated - it will heal. The hormone imbalances that have defined your life for so long are not your destiny. They're symptoms of a terrain that can be restored.

The path is not always easy. It requires commitment, patience, and often significant lifestyle changes. It requires letting go of the quick-fix mentality that drives most of modern medicine. It requires trusting your body's wisdom rather than trying to override it with external interventions.

But the destination - vibrant health, stable energy, clear thinking, emotional balance, and yes, naturally balanced hormones - is worth every step of the journey.

Your hormones are not your enemy. Your body is not broken beyond repair. The imbalance you're experiencing is a symptom - a signal - pointing toward dysfunction that can be addressed. Trust that signal. Follow it to its source. And discover what becomes possible when you stop treating the symptom and start healing the terrain.

Your restoration begins now.

Ready to begin? Scan the code below to complete Dr. Thoma's Dynamic Intake and receive a personalized roadmap for your R.E.S.T.O.R.E. *MILA journey.*

Glossary

A

ATP (Adenosine Triphosphate): The primary energy currency of cells, produced by mitochondria through cellular respiration.

Adrenal Glands: Small glands located on top of each kidney that produce hormones including cortisol, aldosterone, and small amounts of sex hormones.

Aldosterone: A hormone produced by the adrenal glands that regulates sodium and potassium balance, affecting blood pressure and fluid balance.

Amino Acids: The building blocks of proteins, essential for hormone production, enzyme function, and cellular repair.

Antibodies: Proteins produced by the immune system that recognize and bind to foreign substances or, in autoimmune conditions, to the body's own tissues.

Aromatase: An enzyme that converts testosterone to estrogen, particularly active in fat tissue; increased by inflammation and insulin resistance.

Autoimmune: A condition where the body's immune system mistakenly attacks its own healthy cells and tissues.

B

Beta Cells: Specialized cells in the pancreas that produce and secrete insulin in response to blood sugar levels.

Bioidentical Hormones: Synthetic hormones that are chemically identical to those naturally produced by the human body, as opposed to synthetic hormones with different molecular structures.

C

C-Reactive Protein (CRP): A protein produced by the liver in response to inflammation; elevated levels indicate the presence of inflammation in the body.

Cell Danger Response: A cellular survival program activated when cells detect threats, causing mitochondria to shift from energy production to defense mode.

Cell Membrane: The outer boundary of a cell, composed primarily of fatty acids, that controls what enters and exits the cell.

Cholesterol: A waxy lipid molecule essential for cell membrane structure and the raw material for producing all steroid hormones and vitamin D.

Chronic Inflammation: Long-term, low-grade inflammation that persists for months or years, damaging tissues and disrupting normal bodily functions.

Cortisol: A steroid hormone produced by the adrenal glands in response to stress, regulating metabolism, immune function, and inflammation.

D

DHEA (Dehydroepiandrosterone): A precursor hormone produced by the adrenal glands that can be converted into testosterone and estrogen.

Downregulation: The process by which cells decrease the number or sensitivity of receptors in response to chronic exposure to high hormone levels.

E

Endocrine Disruptors: Environmental chemicals that interfere with hormone production, metabolism, or receptor function, mimicking or blocking natural hormones.

Estradiol: The most potent form of estrogen, primarily produced by the ovaries in premenopausal women.

Estrogen: A family of steroid hormones including estradiol, estrone, and estriol that affect reproductive tissues, bone density, brain function, and cardiovascular health.

Estrogen Dominance: A condition where estrogen levels are excessive relative to progesterone, or where estrogen clearance is impaired, causing symptoms even with normal blood levels.

F

Free T3: The unbound, active form of thyroid hormone that is available to enter cells and regulate metabolism.

G

GLP-1 (Glucagon-Like Peptide-1): A hormone produced by the intestines that stimulates insulin secretion, slows stomach emptying, and reduces appetite.

Gut Permeability: Also known as leaky gut, a condition where the intestinal lining becomes compromised, allowing proteins and toxins to enter the bloodstream.

H

Hashimoto's Thyroiditis: An autoimmune condition where the immune system attacks the thyroid gland, causing hypothyroidism.

Hormone Receptor: A protein on or in a cell that binds to specific hormones, allowing the hormone's message to be received and acted upon.

Hyperinsulinemia: Chronically elevated insulin levels in the blood, often preceding type 2 diabetes by years or decades.

Hypothalamus: A region of the brain that monitors hormone levels and sends signals to the pituitary gland to regulate hormone production throughout the body.

Hypothyroidism: A condition where the thyroid gland produces insufficient thyroid hormone, slowing metabolism and causing fatigue, weight gain, and other symptoms.

I

Immune Dysregulation: A state where the immune system is chronically overactive, underactive, or misdirected, attacking the body's own tissues.

Inflammation: The body's protective response to injury or infection, involving immune cells, blood vessels, and molecular mediators.

Insulin: A peptide hormone produced by the pancreas that regulates blood sugar by facilitating glucose uptake into cells.

Insulin Resistance: A condition where cells become less responsive to insulin, requiring higher insulin levels to achieve the same blood sugar control.

L

Leaky Gut: See Gut Permeability.

Lymphatic System: A network of vessels and nodes that drain excess fluid from tissues, transports immune cells, and removes waste products including used hormones.

M

MILA (MY-lah)**:** Mitochondrial-Immune-Lymphatic Axis; the interconnected system of mitochondrial function, immune regulation, and lymphatic drainage that determines overall health.

Mitochondria: Cellular organelles often called the powerhouses of the cell, responsible for producing ATP energy and regulating cellular metabolism.

Mitochondrial Dysfunction: Impaired function of mitochondria leading to reduced energy production and increased oxidative stress.

N

Negative Feedback: A regulatory mechanism where high levels of a hormone signal the body to decrease production, maintaining balance.

O

Omega-3 Fatty Acids: Essential polyunsaturated fats found in fish, flax, and walnuts that reduce inflammation and support cell membrane health.

Omega-6 Fatty Acids: Polyunsaturated fats found in seed oils and processed foods that, in excess, promote inflammation.

Oxidative Stress: An imbalance between free radicals and antioxidants in the body, damaging cells and contributing to chronic disease.

P

Peptide Hormones: Hormones made from chains of amino acids, including insulin, growth hormone, and GLP-1.

Perimenopause: The transitional period before menopause when hormone levels fluctuate, typically beginning in a woman's 40s.

Pituitary Gland: A small gland at the base of the brain, often called the master gland, which produces hormones that control other endocrine glands.

Pregnenolone: The mother hormone produced from cholesterol in the mitochondria, serving as the precursor for all steroid hormones.

Pregnenolone Steal: The phenomenon where chronic stress diverts pregnenolone toward cortisol production, reducing the availability of raw materials for sex hormone production.

Progesterone: A steroid hormone produced mainly by the ovaries after ovulation that balances estrogen, supports pregnancy, and promotes calmness.

R

Receptor Dysfunction: Impaired ability of cellular receptors to receive and respond to hormone signals, causing symptoms of hormone deficiency despite adequate hormone levels.

Reverse T3: An inactive form of thyroid hormone that competes with active T3 for receptors, effectively blocking thyroid function at the cellular level.

S

Steroid Hormones: Hormones derived from cholesterol, including cortisol, testosterone, estrogen, progesterone, and vitamin D.

Supra-physiological: Hormone levels that exceed what the body would naturally produce, often achieved through external hormone supplementation.

T

T3 (Triiodothyronine): The active form of thyroid hormone that regulates metabolic rate and energy production in cells.

T4 (Thyroxine): The storage form of thyroid hormone produced by the thyroid gland, which must be converted to T3 to become active.

TSH (Thyroid Stimulating Hormone): A hormone produced by the pituitary gland that signals the thyroid to produce more thyroid hormone.

Terrain: The internal environment of the body, including mitochondrial function, immune balance, lymphatic flow, and overall cellular health.

Testosterone: The primary male sex hormone, also present in smaller amounts in women, responsible for muscle mass, bone density, energy, and libido.

Thyroid Gland: A butterfly-shaped gland in the neck that produces thyroid hormones controlling metabolism, energy, and body temperature.

Toxic Nine: Nine categories of foods commonly causing inflammation and gut dysfunction: sugar, wheat/gluten, corn, soy, dairy, peanuts, seed oils, alcohol, and chemical additives.

References

[1] Holtorf K. Diagnosis and treatment of hypothyroidism: a patient's perspective. J Restor Med. 2013;2(1):18-32.

[2] Braverman LE, Utiger RD. Werner and Ingbar's The Thyroid: A Fundamental and Clinical Text. 9th ed. Philadelphia, PA: Lippincott Williams & Wilkins; 2005.

[3] Wiersinga WM. Paradigm shifts in thyroid hormone replacement therapies for hypothyroidism. Nat Rev Endocrinol. 2014;10(3):164-174.

[4] Hoermann R, Midgley JE, Larisch R, Dietrich JW. Homeostatic control of the thyroid-pituitary axis: perspectives for diagnosis and treatment. Front Endocrinol. 2015;6:177.

[5] Mullur R, Liu YY, Brent GA. Thyroid hormone regulation of metabolism. Physiol Rev. 2014;94(2):355-382.

[6] Pieczenik SR, Neustadt J. Mitochondrial dysfunction and molecular pathways of disease. Exp Mol Pathol. 2007;83(1):84-92.

[7] Simopoulos AP. The importance of the ratio of omega-6/omega-3 essential fatty acids. Biomed Pharmacother. 2002;56(8):365-379.

[8] Chrousos GP. Stress and disorders of the stress system. Nat Rev Endocrinol. 2009;5(7):374-381.

[9] Veldhuis JD, Roelfsema F, Iranmanesh A, Carroll BJ, Keenan DM, Pincus SM. Basal, pulsatile, entropic, and 24-hour rhythmic features of secondary adrenal failure. Am J

Physiol Regul Integr Comp Physiol. 2012;303(10):R1049-R1063.

[10] Corona G, Rastrelli G, Morgentaler A, Sforza A, Mannucci E, Maggi M. Meta-analysis of results of testosterone therapy on sexual function based on international index of erectile function scores. Eur Urol. 2017;72(6):1000-1011.

[11] Hyman M. The UltraMind Solution: Fix Your Broken Brain by Healing Your Body First. New York, NY: Scribner; 2009.

[12] Saper CB, Lowell BB. The hypothalamus. Curr Biol. 2014;24(23):R1111-R1116.

[13] Miller WL. Steroid hormone synthesis in mitochondria. Mol Cell Endocrinol. 2013;379(1-2):62-73.

[14] Kronenberg H, Melmed S, Polonsky K, Larsen PR. Williams Textbook of Endocrinology. 12th ed. Philadelphia, PA: Saunders; 2011.

[15] Boron WF, Boulpaep EL. Medical Physiology. 3rd ed. Philadelphia, PA: Elsevier; 2017.

[16] Beato M, Klug J. Steroid hormone receptors: an update. Hum Reprod Update. 2000;6(3):225-236.

[17] Maninger N, Wolkowitz OM, Reus VI, Epel ES, Mellon SH. Neurobiological and neuropsychiatric effects of dehydroepiandrosterone (DHEA) and DHEA sulfate (DHEAS). Front Neuroendocrinol. 2009;30(1):65-91.

[18] Cheng SY, Leonard JL, Davis PJ. Molecular aspects of thyroid hormone actions. Endocr Rev. 2010;31(2):139-170.

[19] Tsigos C, Chrousos GP. Hypothalamic-pituitary-adrenal axis, neuroendocrine factors and stress. J Psychosom Res. 2002;53(4):865-871.

[20] Sapolsky RM, Romero LM, Munck AU. How do glucocorticoids influence stress responses? Integrating permissive, suppressive, stimulatory, and preparative actions. Endocr Rev. 2000;21(1):55-89.

[21] DeFronzo RA, Tripathy D. Skeletal muscle insulin resistance is the primary defect in type 2 diabetes. Diabetes Care. 2009;32 Suppl 2:S157-S163.

[22] Fries E, Hesse J, Hellhammer J, Hellhammer DH. A new view on hypocortisolism. Psychoneuroendocrinology. 2005;30(10):1010-1016.

[23] Bhasin S, Brito JP, Cunningham GR, et al. Testosterone therapy in men with hypogonadism: an Endocrine Society clinical practice guideline. J Clin Endocrinol Metab. 2018;103(5):1715-1744.

[24] Davis SR, Wahlin-Jacobsen S. Testosterone in women - the clinical significance. Lancet Diabetes Endocrinol. 2015;3(12):980-992.

[25] McEwen BS. Physiology and neurobiology of stress and adaptation: central role of the brain. Physiol Rev. 2007;87(3):873-904.

[26] Khosla S, Monroe DG. Regulation of bone metabolism by sex steroids. Cold Spring Harb Perspect Med. 2018;8(1):a031211.

[27] Stuenkel CA, Davis SR, Gompel A, et al. Treatment of symptoms of the menopause: an Endocrine Society clinical

practice guideline. J Clin Endocrinol Metab. 2015;100(11):3975-4011.

[28] Brinton RD. Estrogen-induced plasticity from cells to circuits: predictions for cognitive function. Trends Pharmacol Sci. 2009;30(4):212-222.

[29] Naviaux RK. Metabolic features of the cell danger response. Mitochondrion. 2014;16:7-17.

[30] Wallace DC. A mitochondrial paradigm of metabolic and degenerative diseases, aging, and cancer: a dawn for evolutionary medicine. Annu Rev Genet. 2005;39:359-407.

[31] Boelen A, Kwakkel J, Fliers E. Beyond low plasma T3: local thyroid hormone metabolism during inflammation and infection. Endocr Rev. 2011;32(5):670-693.

[32] Aspelund A, Robciuc MR, Karber S, et al. Lymphatic system in cardiovascular medicine. Circ Res. 2016;118(3):515-530.

[33] Moore JE Jr, Bertram CD. Lymphatic System Flows. Annu Rev Fluid Mech. 2018;50:459-482.

[34] Mortimer PS, Rockson SG. New developments in clinical aspects of lymphatic disease. J Clin Invest. 2014;124(3):915-921.

[35] Straub RH. The complex role of estrogens in inflammation. Endocr Rev. 2007;28(5):521-574.

[36] Simpson ER, Brown KA. Minireview: obesity and breast cancer: a tale of inflammation and dysregulated metabolism. Mol Endocrinol. 2013;27(5):715-725.

[37] Chung HY, Cesari M, Anton S, et al. Molecular inflammation: underpinnings of aging and age-related diseases. Ageing Res Rev. 2009;8(1):18-30.

[38] Mangelsdorf DJ, Thummel C, Beato M, et al. The nuclear receptor superfamily: the second decade. Cell. 1995;83(6):835-839.

[39] Liao S, Cheng G, Conner DA, et al. Impaired lymphatic contraction associated with immunosuppression. Proc Natl Acad Sci USA. 2011;108(46):18784-18789.

[40] Hulbert AJ, Turner N, Storlien LH, Else PL. Dietary fats and membrane function: implications for metabolism and disease. Biol Rev Camb Philos Soc. 2005;80(1):155-169.

[41] Zhu BT, Conney AH. Functional role of estrogen metabolism in target cells: review and perspectives. Carcinogenesis. 1998;19(1):1-27.

[42] Wallace DC. Mitochondrial DNA mutations in disease and aging. Environ Mol Mutagen. 2010;51(5):440-450.

[43] de Heredia FP, Gomez-Martinez S, Marcos A. Obesity, inflammation and the immune system. Proc Nutr Soc. 2012;71(2):332-338.

[44] Hotamisligil GS. Inflammation and metabolic disorders. Nature. 2006;444(7121):860-867.

[45] Bradlow HL, Telang NT, Sepkovic DW, Osborne MP. 2-hydroxyestrone: the 'good' estrogen. J Endocrinol. 1996;150 Suppl:S259-S265.

[46] Davis PJ, Goglia F, Leonard JL. Nongenomic actions of thyroid hormone. Nat Rev Endocrinol. 2016;12(2):111-121.

[47] Psarra AM, Sekeris CE. Steroid and thyroid hormone receptors in mitochondria. IUBMB Life. 2008;60(4):210-223.

[48] Aranda A, Pascual A. Nuclear hormone receptors and gene expression. Physiol Rev. 2001;81(3):1269-1304.

[49] Mangelsdorf DJ, Evans RM. The RXR heterodimers and orphan receptors. Cell. 1995;83(6):841-850.

[50] Koenig RJ. Thyroid hormone receptor coactivators and corepressors. Thyroid. 1998;8(8):703-713.

[51] Brent GA. Mechanisms of thyroid hormone action. J Clin Invest. 2012;122(9):3035-3043.

[52] Vandenberg LN, Colborn T, Hayes TB, et al. Hormones and endocrine-disrupting chemicals: low-dose effects and non-monotonic dose responses. Endocr Rev. 2012;33(3):378-455.

[53] Kenakin T. Receptor theory in pharmacology. Trends Pharmacol Sci. 2004;25(4):186-192.

[54] Calder PC. Omega-3 fatty acids and inflammatory processes: from molecules to man. Biochem Soc Trans. 2017;45(5):1105-1115.

[55] Fasano A. Zonulin, regulation of tight junctions, and autoimmune diseases. Ann N Y Acad Sci. 2012;1258(1):25-33.

[56] Caturegli P, De Remigis A, Rose NR. Hashimoto thyroiditis: clinical and diagnostic criteria. Autoimmun Rev. 2014;13(4-5):391-397.

[57] Duntas LH. Environmental factors and thyroid autoimmunity. Ann Endocrinol (Paris). 2011;72(2):108-113.

[58] McLeod DS, Cooper DS. The incidence and prevalence of thyroid autoimmunity. Endocrine. 2012;42(2):252-265.

[59] Tomer Y, Huber A. The etiology of autoimmune thyroid disease: a story of genes and environment. J Autoimmun. 2009;32(3-4):231-239.

[60] Sfriso P, Ghirardello A, Botsios C, et al. Infections and autoimmunity: the multifaceted relationship. J Leukoc Biol. 2010;87(3):385-395.

[61] Fasano A. Leaky gut and autoimmune diseases. Clin Rev Allergy Immunol. 2012;42(1):71-78.

[62] Brent GA. Environmental exposures and autoimmune thyroid disease. Thyroid. 2010;20(7):755-761.

[63] Hollowell JG, Staehling NW, Flanders WD, et al. Serum TSH, T(4), and thyroid antibodies in the United States population (1988 to 1994): National Health and Nutrition Examination Survey (NHANES III). J Clin Endocrinol Metab. 2002;87(2):489-499.

[64] Wilding JPH, Batterham RL, Calanna S, et al. Once-weekly semaglutide in adults with overweight or obesity. N Engl J Med. 2021;384(11):989-1002.

[65] Mazokopakis EE, Kotsiris DA. Hashimoto's autoimmune thyroiditis and vitamin D deficiency. Current aspects. Hell J Nucl Med. 2014;17(1):37-40.

[66] Chaudhary S, Dutta D, Kumar M, et al. Vitamin D supplementation reduces thyroid peroxidase antibody levels in patients with autoimmune thyroid disease: an open-labeled randomized controlled trial. Indian J Endocrinol Metab. 2016;20(3):391-398.

[67] DeFronzo RA, Ferrannini E, Groop L, et al. Type 2 diabetes mellitus. Nat Rev Dis Primers. 2015;1:15019.

[68] Petersen MC, Shulman GI. Mechanisms of insulin action and insulin resistance. Physiol Rev. 2018;98(4):2133-2223.

[69] Bianco AC, Salvatore D, Gereben B, Berry MJ, Larsen PR. Biochemistry, cellular and molecular biology, and physiological roles of the iodothyronine selenodeiodinases. Endocr Rev. 2002;23(1):38-89.

[70] Drucker DJ, Nauck MA. The incretin system: glucagon-like peptide-1 receptor agonists and dipeptidyl peptidase-4 inhibitors in type 2 diabetes. Lancet. 2006;368(9548):1696-1705.

[71] Jastreboff AM, Aronne LJ, Ahmad NN, et al. Tirzepatide once weekly for the treatment of obesity. N Engl J Med. 2022;387(3):205-216.

[72] Szendroedi J, Phielix E, Roden M. The role of mitochondria in insulin resistance and type 2 diabetes mellitus. Nat Rev Endocrinol. 2012;8(2):92-103.

[73] Nicolaides NC, Charmandari E, Chrousos GP, Kino T. Circadian endocrine rhythms: the hypothalamic-pituitary-adrenal axis and its actions. Ann N Y Acad Sci. 2014;1318:71-80.

[74] Charmandari E, Tsigos C, Chrousos G. Endocrinology of the stress response. Annu Rev Physiol. 2005;67:259-284.

[75] McEwen BS. Protective and damaging effects of stress mediators: central role of the brain. Dialogues Clin Neurosci. 2006;8(4):367-381.

[76] Hannibal KE, Bishop MD. Chronic stress, cortisol dysfunction, and pain: a psychoneuroendocrine rationale for stress management in pain rehabilitation. Phys Ther. 2014;94(12):1816-1825.

[77] Cadegiani FA, Kater CE. Adrenal fatigue does not exist: a systematic review. BMC Endocr Disord. 2016;16(1):48.

[78] Wilson JL. Adrenal Fatigue: The 21st Century Stress Syndrome. Petaluma, CA: Smart Publications; 2001.

[79] Golomb BA, Evans MA. Statin adverse effects: a review of the literature and evidence for a mitochondrial mechanism. Am J Cardiovasc Drugs. 2008;8(6):373-418.

[80] Miller WL, Auchus RJ. The molecular biology, biochemistry, and physiology of human steroidogenesis and its disorders. Endocr Rev. 2011;32(1):81-151.

[81] Mowat AM, Agace WW. Regional specialization within the intestinal immune system. Nat Rev Immunol. 2014;14(10):667-685.

[82] Leproult R, Copinschi G, Buxton O, Van Cauter E. Sleep loss results in an elevation of cortisol levels the next evening. Sleep. 1997;20(10):865-870.

[83] Chandrasekhar K, Kapoor J, Anishetty S. A prospective, randomized double-blind, placebo-controlled study of safety and efficacy of a high-concentration full-spectrum extract of ashwagandha root in reducing stress and anxiety in adults. Indian J Psychol Med. 2012;34(3):255-262.

[84] Lovallo WR, Whitsett TL, al'Absi M, Sung BH, Vincent AS, Wilson MF. Caffeine stimulation of cortisol secretion across the waking hours in relation to caffeine intake levels. Psychosom Med. 2005;67(5):734-739.

[85] Hamalainen EK, Adlercreutz H, Puska P, Pietinen P. Decrease of serum total and free testosterone during a low-fat high-fibre diet. J Steroid Biochem. 1984;20(1):459-464.

[86] Finkelstein JS, Lee H, Burnett-Bowie SA, et al. Gonadal steroids and body composition, strength, and sexual function in men. N Engl J Med. 2013;369(11):1011-1022.

[87] Davis SR, Moreau M, Kroll R, et al. Testosterone for low libido in postmenopausal women not taking estrogen. N Engl J Med. 2008;359(19):2005-2017.

[88] Wierman ME, Arlt W, Basson R, et al. Androgen therapy in women: a reappraisal: an Endocrine Society clinical practice guideline. J Clin Endocrinol Metab. 2014;99(10):3489-3510.

[89] Rossouw JE, Anderson GL, Prentice RL, et al. Risks and benefits of estrogen plus progestin in healthy postmenopausal women: principal results from the Women's Health Initiative randomized controlled trial. JAMA. 2002;288(3):321-333.

[90] Manson JE, Chlebowski RT, Stefanick ML, et al. Menopausal hormone therapy and health outcomes during the intervention and extended poststopping phases of the Women's Health Initiative randomized trials. JAMA. 2013;310(13):1353-1368.

[91] Sarrel PM, Njike VY, Vinante V, Katz DL. The mortality toll of estrogen avoidance: an analysis of excess deaths among hysterectomized women aged 50 to 59 years. Am J Public Health. 2013;103(9):1583-1588.

[92] Hodis HN, Mack WJ, Henderson VW, et al. Vascular effects of early versus late postmenopausal treatment with estradiol. N Engl J Med. 2016;374(13):1221-1231.

[93] Simpson ER. Sources of estrogen and their importance. J Steroid Biochem Mol Biol. 2003;86(3-5):225-230.

[94] Shifren JL, Gass ML. The North American Menopause Society recommendations for clinical care of midlife women. Menopause. 2014;21(10):1038-1062.

[95] Layman LC. The genetic basis of female reproductive disorders: etiology and clinical testing. Mol Cell Endocrinol. 2013;370(1-2):138-148.

[96] Travison TG, Araujo AB, O'Donnell AB, Kupelian V, McKinlay JB. A population-level decline in serum testosterone levels in American men. J Clin Endocrinol Metab. 2007;92(1):196-202.

[97] Diamanti-Kandarakis E, Bourguignon JP, Giudice LC, et al. Endocrine-disrupting chemicals: an Endocrine Society scientific statement. Endocr Rev. 2009;30(4):293-342.

[98] Dunn JF, Nisula BC, Rodbard D. Transport of steroid hormones: binding of 21 endogenous steroids to both testosterone-binding globulin and corticosteroid-binding globulin in human plasma. J Clin Endocrinol Metab. 1981;53(1):58-68.

[99] Bland JS. The Disease Delusion: Conquering the Causes of Chronic Illness for a Healthier, Longer, and Happier Life. New York, NY: Harper Wave; 2014.

[100] Gore AC, Chappell VA, Fenton SE, et al. EDC-2: The Endocrine Society's second scientific statement on endocrine-disrupting chemicals. Endocr Rev. 2015;36(6):E1-E150.

[101] Tilbrook AJ, Turner AI, Clarke IJ. Effects of stress on reproduction in non-rodent mammals: the role of

glucocorticoids and sex differences. Rev Reprod. 2000;5(2):105-113.

[102] Menon KMJ, Menon B. Structure, function and regulation of gonadotropin receptors - a perspective. Mol Cell Endocrinol. 2012;356(1-2):88-97.

[103] Stanczyk FZ, Hapgood JP, Winer S, Mishell DR Jr. Progestogens used in postmenopausal hormone therapy: differences in their pharmacological properties, intracellular actions, and clinical effects. Endocr Rev. 2013;34(2):171-208.

[104] Shuster LT, Rhodes DJ, Gostout BS, Grossardt BR, Rocca WA. Premature menopause or early menopause: long-term health consequences. Maturitas. 2010;65(2):161-166.

[105] Rocca WA, Grossardt BR, Shuster LT. Oophorectomy, estrogen, and dementia: a 2014 update. Mol Cell Endocrinol. 2014;389(1-2):7-12.

[106] Basaria S, Coviello AD, Travison TG, et al. Adverse events associated with testosterone administration. N Engl J Med. 2010;363(2):109-122.

[107] Dantzer R, O'Connor JC, Freund GG, Johnson RW, Kelley KW. From inflammation to sickness and depression: when the immune system subjugates the brain. Nat Rev Neurosci. 2008;9(1):46-56.

[108] Saper CB, Scammell TE, Lu J. Hypothalamic regulation of sleep and circadian rhythms. Nature. 2005;437(7063):1257-1263.

[109] Porges SW. The polyvagal theory: phylogenetic substrates of a social nervous system. Int J Psychophysiol. 2001;42(2):123-146.

[110] Dalle-Donne I, Rossi R, Colombo R, Giustarini D, Milzani A. Biomarkers of oxidative damage in human disease. Clin Chem. 2006;52(4):601-623.

[111] Fernstrom JD, Fernstrom MH. Tyrosine, phenylalanine, and catecholamine synthesis and function in the brain. J Nutr. 2007;137(6 Suppl 1):1539S-1547S.

[112] Hodges RE, Minich DM. Modulation of metabolic detoxification pathways using foods and food-derived components: a scientific review with clinical application. J Nutr Metab. 2015;2015:760689.

[113] Sies H, Jones DP. Reactive oxygen species (ROS) as pleiotropic physiological signalling agents. Nat Rev Mol Cell Biol. 2020;21(7):363-383.

[114] Liew SC, Gupta ED. Methylenetetrahydrofolate reductase (MTHFR) C677T polymorphism: epidemiology, metabolism and the associated diseases. Eur J Med Genet. 2015;58(1):1-10.

[115] Koh A, De Vadder F, Kovatcheva-Datchary P, Backhed F. From dietary fiber to host physiology: short-chain fatty acids as key bacterial metabolites. Cell. 2016;166(6):1332-1345.

[116] Plottel CS, Blaser MJ. Microbiome and malignancy. Cell Host Microbe. 2011;10(4):324-335.

[117] McEwen BS. Stress, adaptation, and disease: allostasis and allostatic load. Ann N Y Acad Sci. 1998;840:33-44.

[118] Chikly B. Silent Waves: Theory and Practice of Lymph Drainage Therapy. 2nd ed. Scottsdale, AZ: IHH Publishing; 2004.

[119] Genuis SJ. Elimination of persistent toxicants from the human body. Hum Exp Toxicol. 2011;30(1):3-18.

[120] Sears ME, Kerr KJ, Bray RI. Arsenic, cadmium, lead, and mercury in sweat: a systematic review. J Environ Public Health. 2012;2012:184745.

[121] Mesnage R, Clair E, Gress S, Then C, Szekacs A, Seralini GE. Cytotoxicity on human cells of Cry1Ab and Cry1Ac Bt insecticidal toxins alone or with a glyphosate-based herbicide. J Appl Toxicol. 2013;33(7):695-699.

[122] Brooke-Taylor S, Dwyer K, Woodford K, Kost N. Systematic review of the gastrointestinal effects of A1 compared with A2 beta-casein. Nutrients. 2017;9(2):739.

[123] DiNicolantonio JJ, O'Keefe JH. Omega-6 vegetable oils as a driver of coronary heart disease: the oxidized linoleic acid hypothesis. Open Heart. 2018;5(2):e000898.

[124] Kessler R. Studies begin to clarify health risks from common chemical. Environ Health Perspect. 2015;123(2):A42.

[125] Shields JW. Lymph, lymph glands, and homeostasis. Lymphology. 1992;25(4):147-153.

[126] Olszewski WL. Contractility patterns of normal and pathologically changed human lymphatics. Ann N Y Acad Sci. 2002;979:52-63.

[127] Ballatori N, Krance SM, Notenboom S, Shi S, Tieu K, Hammond CL. Glutathione dysregulation and the etiology and progression of human diseases. Biol Chem. 2009;390(3):191-214.

[128] Lustig RH, Schmidt LA, Brindis CD. Public health: the toxic truth about sugar. Nature. 2012;482(7383):27-29.

[129] Vojdani A. Lectins, agglutinins, and their roles in autoimmune reactivities. Altern Ther Health Med. 2015;21 Suppl 1:46-51.

[130] Johnson RK, Appel LJ, Brands M, et al. Dietary sugars intake and cardiovascular health: a scientific statement from the American Heart Association. Circulation. 2009;120(11):1011-1020.

[131] Doerge DR, Sheehan DM. Goitrogenic and estrogenic activity of soy isoflavones. Environ Health Perspect. 2002;110 Suppl 3:349-353.

[132] Woodford K. Devil in the Milk: Illness, Health and the Politics of A1 and A2 Milk. White River Junction, VT: Chelsea Green Publishing; 2009.

[133] Pal S, Woodford K, Kukuljan S, Ho S. Milk intolerance, beta- casein and lactose. Nutrients. 2015;7(9):7285-7297.

[134] Strosnider H, Azziz-Baumgartner E, Banziger M, et al. Workgroup report: public health strategies for reducing aflatoxin exposure in developing countries. Environ Health Perspect. 2006;114(12):1898-1903.

[135] Vermeulen A, Kaufman JM, Goemaere S, van Pottelberg I. Estradiol in elderly men. Aging Male. 2002;5(2):98-102.

[136] Ramsden CE, Zamora D, Leelarthaepin B, et al. Use of dietary linoleic acid for secondary prevention of coronary heart disease and death: evaluation of recovered data from the Sydney Diet Heart Study and updated meta- analysis. BMJ. 2013;346:e8707.

[137] Blasbalg TL, Hibbeln JR, Ramsden CE, Majchrzak SF, Rawlings RR. Changes in consumption of omega-3 and

omega-6 fatty acids in the United States during the 20th century. Am J Clin Nutr. 2011;93(5):950-962.

[138] Bode C, Bode JC. Alcohol's role in gastrointestinal tract disorders. Alcohol Health Res World. 1997;21(1):76-83.

[139] Suez J, Korem T, Zeevi D, et al. Artificial sweeteners induce glucose intolerance by altering the gut microbiota. Nature. 2014;514(7521):181-186.

[140] Arnold LE, Lofthouse N, Hurt E. Artificial food colors and attention-deficit/hyperactivity symptoms: conclusions to dye for. Neurotherapeutics. 2012;9(3):599-609.

[141] Wild CP, Gong YY. Mycotoxins and human disease: a largely ignored global health issue. Carcinogenesis. 2010;31(1):71-82.

[142] Blasbalg TL, Hibbeln JR, Ramsden CE, et al. Changes in consumption of omega-3 and omega-6 fatty acids in the United States during the 20th century. Am J Clin Nutr. 2011;93(5):950-962.

[143] Mayer EA. Gut feelings: the emerging biology of gut-brain communication. Nat Rev Neurosci. 2011;12(8):453-466.

[144] Sonnenburg ED, Sonnenburg JL. Starving our microbial self: the deleterious consequences of a diet deficient in microbiota-accessible carbohydrates. Cell Metab. 2014;20(5):779-786.

[145] David LA, Maurice CF, Carmody RN, et al. Diet rapidly and reproducibly alters the human gut microbiome. Nature. 2014;505(7484):559-563.

[146] Le Chatelier E, Nielsen T, Qin J, et al. Richness of human gut microbiome correlates with metabolic markers. Nature. 2013;500(7464):541-546.

[147] Mattson MP, Longo VD, Harvie M. Impact of intermittent fasting on health and disease processes. Ageing Res Rev. 2017;39:46-58.

[148] de Cabo R, Mattson MP. Effects of intermittent fasting on health, aging, and disease. N Engl J Med. 2019;381(26):2541-2551.

[149] Daley CA, Abbott A, Doyle PS, Nader GA, Larson S. A review of fatty acid profiles and antioxidant content in grass-fed and grain-fed beef. Nutr J. 2010;9:10.

[150] Patterson RE, Sears DD. Metabolic effects of intermittent fasting. Annu Rev Nutr. 2017;37:371-393.

[151] Sutton EF, Beyl R, Early KS, Cefalu WT, Ravussin E, Peterson CM. Early time-restricted feeding improves insulin sensitivity, blood pressure, and oxidative stress Metab. 2018;27(6):1212-1221.e3.

[152] Wilkinson MJ, Manoogian ENC, Zadourian A, et al. Ten-hour time-restricted eating reduces weight, blood pressure, and atherogenic lipids in patients with metabolic syndrome. Cell Metab. 2020;31(1):92-104.e5.

[153] Levine B, Kroemer G. Biological functions of autophagy genes: a disease perspective. Cell. 2019;176(1-2):11-42.

[154] Bray GA, Popkin BM. Dietary sugar and body weight: have we reached a crisis in the epidemic of obesity and metabolic diseases? Diabetes Care. 2014;37(4):950-956.

[155] Dinarello CA. Historical insights into cytokines. Eur J Immunol. 2007;37 Suppl 1:S34-S45.

[156] Sakaguchi S, Yamaguchi T, Nomura T, Ono M. Regulatory T cells and immune tolerance. Cell. 2008;133(5):775-787.

[157] Fairweather D, Rose NR. Women and autoimmune diseases. Emerg Infect Dis. 2004;10(11):2005-2011.

[158] Serhan CN. Pro-resolving lipid mediators are leads for resolution physiology. Nature. 2014;510(7503):92-101.

[159] Gleeson M, Bishop NC, Stensel DJ, Lindley MR, Mastana SS, Nimmo MA. The anti-inflammatory effects of exercise: mechanisms and implications for the prevention and treatment of disease. Nat Rev Immunol. 2011;11(9):607-615.

[160] Besedovsky L, Lange T, Born J. Sleep and immune function. Pflugers Arch. 2012;463(1):121-137.

[161] Segerstrom SC, Miller GE. Psychological stress and the human immune system: a meta-analytic study of 30 years of inquiry. Psychol Bull. 2004;130(4):601-630.

[162] Cole SW, Hawkley LC, Arevalo JM, Sung CY, Rose RM, Cacioppo JT. Social regulation of gene expression in human leukocytes. Genome Biol. 2007;8(9):R189.

[163] Ueberall MA, Mueller-Schwefe GH, Wigand R, Essner U. Efficacy, tolerability, and safety of an oral enzyme Clin J Pain. 2016;32(12):1032-1042.

[164] Aggarwal BB, Harikumar KB. Potential therapeutic effects of curcumin, the anti-inflammatory agent, against neurodegenerative, cardiovascular, pulmonary, metabolic,

autoimmune and neoplastic diseases. Int J Biochem Cell Biol. 2009;41(1):40-59.

[165] Dröge W, Breitkreutz R. Glutathione and immune function. Proc Nutr Soc. 2000;59(4):595-600.

[166] Vander Heiden MG, Cantley LC, Thompson CB. Understanding the Warburg effect: the metabolic requirements of cell proliferation. Science. 2009;324(5930):1029-1033.

[167] Papadopoulos V, Miller WL. Role of mitochondria in steroidogenesis. Best Pract Res Clin Endocrinol Metab. 2012;26(6):771-790.

[168] Guo Y, Jolly RA, Halstead BW, et al. Transcriptomic and metabolomic analysis of liver function. Drug Metab Dispos. 2016;44(7):1043-1052.

[169] Bianco AC, Kim BW. Deiodinases: implications of the local control of thyroid hormone action. J Clin Invest. 2006;116(10):2571-2579.

[170] Jornayvaz FR, Shulman GI. Regulation of mitochondrial biogenesis. Essays Biochem. 2010;47:69-84.

[171] Cannon B, Nedergaard J. Brown adipose tissue: function and physiological significance. Physiol Rev. 2004;84(1):277-359.

[172] Laukkanen JA, Laukkanen T, Kunutsor SK. Cardiovascular and other health benefits of sauna bathing: a review of the evidence. Mayo Clin Proc. 2018;93(8):1111-1121.

[173] Kirkland JL, Tchkonia T. Senolytic drugs: from discovery to translation. J Intern Med. 2020;288(5):518-536.

[174] Pekala J, Patkowska-Sokola B, Bodkowski R, et al. L-carnitine - metabolic functions and meaning in humans life. Curr Drug Metab. 2011;12(7):667-678.

[175] Littarru GP, Tiano L. Bioenergetic and antioxidant properties of coenzyme Q10: recent developments. Mol Biotechnol. 2007;37(1):31-37.

[176] Depeint F, Bruce WR, Bhathena SJ, et al. Mitochondrial function and toxicity: role of the B vitamin family on mitochondrial energy metabolism. Chem Biol Interact. 2006;163(1-2):94-112.

[177] Pilchova I, Klacanova K, Tatarkova Z, Kaplan P, Bhide M. The involvement of Mg2+ in regulation of cellular and mitochondrial functions. Oxid Med Cell Longev. 2017;2017:6797460.

[178] Mari M, Morales A, Colell A, Garcia-Ruiz C, Fernandez-Checa JC. Mitochondrial glutathione, a key survival antioxidant. Antioxid Redox Signal. 2009;11(11):2685-2700.

[179] Gomez-Pinilla F. Brain foods: the effects of nutrients on brain function. Nat Rev Neurosci. 2008;9(7):568-578.

[180] Raichle ME, Gusnard DA. Appraising the brain's energy budget. Proc Natl Acad Sci U S A. 2002;99(16):10237-10239.

[181] Jessen NA, Munk AS, Lundgaard I, Bhargava P. The glymphatic system: a beginner's guide. Neurochem Res. 2015;40(12):2583-2599.

[182] Xie L, Kang H, Xu Q, et al. Sleep drives metabolite clearance from the adult brain. Science. 2013;342(6156):373-377.

[183] Breit S, Kupferberg A, Rogler G, Hasler G. Vagus nerve as modulator of the brain-gut axis in psychiatric and inflammatory disorders. Front Psychiatry. 2018;9:44.

[184] Walker M. Why We Sleep: Unlocking the Power of Sleep and Dreams. New York, NY: Scribner; 2017.

[185] Lee H, Xie L, Yu M, et al. The effect of body posture on brain glymphatic transport. J Neurosci. 2015;35(31):11034-11044.

[186] Gerritsen RJS, Band GPH. Breath of life: the respiratory vagal stimulation model of contemplative activity. Front Hum Neurosci. 2018;12:397.

[187] Merzenich MM, Van Vleet TM, Nahum M. Brain plasticity- based therapeutics. Front Hum Neurosci. 2014;8:385.

[188] Bratman GN, Hamilton JP, Hahn KS, Daily GC, Gross JJ. Nature experience reduces rumination and subgenual prefrontal cortex activation. Proc Natl Acad Sci U S A. 2015;112(28):8567-8572.

[189] Kok BE, Coffey KA, Cohn MA, et al. How positive emotions build physical health: perceived positive social connections account for the upward spiral between 2013;24(7):1123-1132.

[190] Slutsky I, Abumaria N, Wu LJ, et al. Enhancement of learning and memory by elevating brain magnesium. Neuron. 2010;65(2):165-177.

[191] Dringen R. Metabolism and functions of glutathione in brain. Prog Neurobiol. 2000;62(6):649-671.

[192] Spalding KL, Bhardwaj RD, Buchholz BA, Druid H, Frisen J. Retrospective birth dating of cells in humans. Cell. 2005;122(1):133-143.

[193] Phillips SM, Van Loon LJ. Dietary protein for athletes: from requirements to optimum adaptation. J Sports Sci. 2011;29 Suppl 1:S29-S38.

[194] McEwen BS. Stressed or stressed out: what is the difference? J Psychiatry Neurosci. 2005;30(5):315-318.

[195] Pedersen BK, Saltin B. Exercise as medicine - evidence for prescribing exercise as therapy in 26 different chronic diseases. Scand J Med Sci Sports. 2015;25 Suppl 3:1-72.

[196] Fairfield KM, Fletcher RH. Vitamins for chronic disease prevention in adults: scientific review. JAMA. 2002;287(23):3116-3126.

[197] Holick MF. Vitamin D deficiency. N Engl J Med. 2007;357(3):266-281.

[198] Price C, Hooven C. Interoceptive awareness skills for emotion regulation: theory and approach of mindful awareness in body-oriented therapy (MABT). Front Psychol. 2018;9:798.

[199] Longo VD, Mattson MP. Fasting: molecular mechanisms and clinical applications. Cell Metab. 2014;19(2):181-192.

www.ingramcontent.com/pod-product-compliance
Lightning Source LLC
Chambersburg PA
CBHW071425230926
51846CB00001B/121
9781971449067